PRAISE FOR *FEEL BETTER IN 5*

"Rangan's easy, common-sense plan can help everyone live a happier, healthier life."

—JAMIE OLIVER, CHEF, RESTAURATEUR, AND BESTSELLING AUTHOR

"One of the best habit change programs I have ever come across. Deceptively simple but remarkably effective."

—BJ FOGG, AUTHOR OF *TINY HABITS* AND PROFESSOR AT STANFORD UNIVERSITY

"One of the most influential doctors in the country."

—CHRIS EVANS, ENGLISH RADIO DJ AND TV PRESENTER

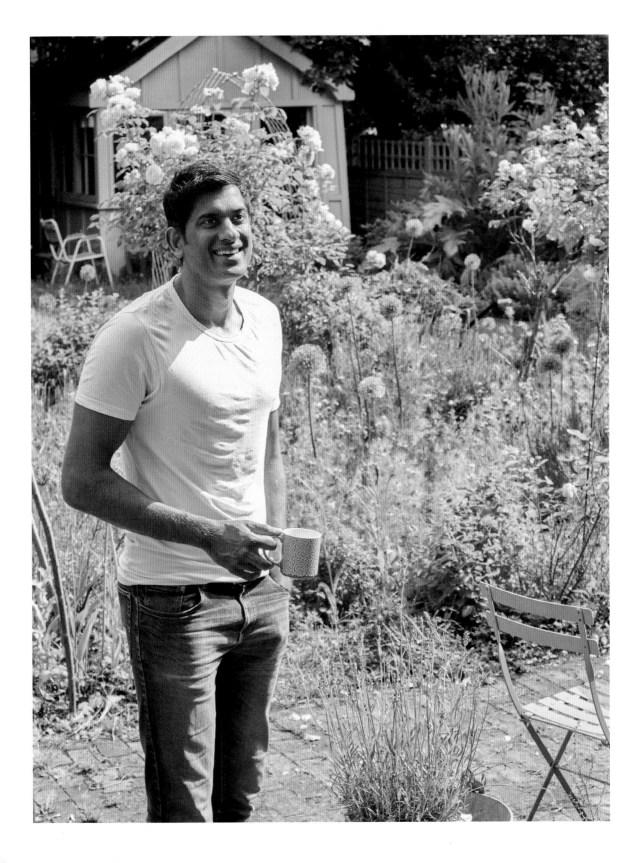

DR. RANGAN CHATTERJEE

FEEL BETTER IN 5

YOUR DAILY PLAN TO FEEL GREAT FOR LIFE

PHOTOGRAPHY BY CLARE WINFIELD

BENBELLA

BenBella Books, Inc.
Dallas, TX

Feel Better in 5 copyright © 2020 by Rangan Chatterjee
Photography copyright © 2020 Clare Winfield
Cover design by Penguin Random House UK and BenBella Books
Interior design by Penguin Random House UK

BENBELLA

BenBella Books, Inc.
10440 N. Central Expressway
Suite 800
Dallas, TX 75231
www.benbellabooks.com
Send feedback to feedback@benbellabooks.com

BenBella is a federally registered trademark.

Printed in the United States of America
10 9 8 7 6 5 4 3 2 1

Originally published by Penguin Random House UK

Library of Congress Cataloging-in-Publication Data is available upon request.
ISBN 9781950665686 (trade paperback)
ISBN 9781950665723 (ebook)

Distributed to the trade by Two Rivers Distribution, an Ingram brand
www.tworiversdistribution.com

TO MY MOTHER,
THANKS FOR EVERYTHING.

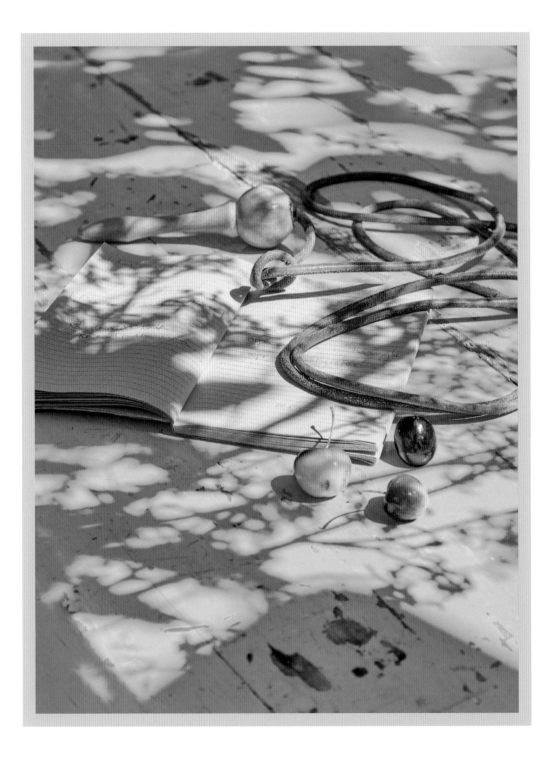

CONTENTS

Welcome to Success **9** | Your Life Can Be Medicine **15**

Changing Your Life by Changing the Journey **19** | We Are Our Habits **22**

The Ripple Effect **25** | Six Tips for Making Changes That Stick **26**

How to Do the Plan **38** | Key for Benefits **40** | How to Choose Your Health
Snacks **42** | How to Get Less . . . **45** | How to Get More . . . **51**

1
MIND

DOWNLOAD
65

NATURE
74

FLOW
84

BREATHE
92

NOURISH
102

2
BODY

STRENGTH
116

SWEAT
134

PLAY
154

BALANCE
166

RESTORE
188

3
HEART

CONNECT
212

FORGIVE
226

CELEBRATE
234

Conclusion: Toothbrushing for Everything Else **259**

Frequently Asked Questions **264** | Further Resources **266**

Acknowledgments **267** | Health Snacks Index **268** | Index **269**

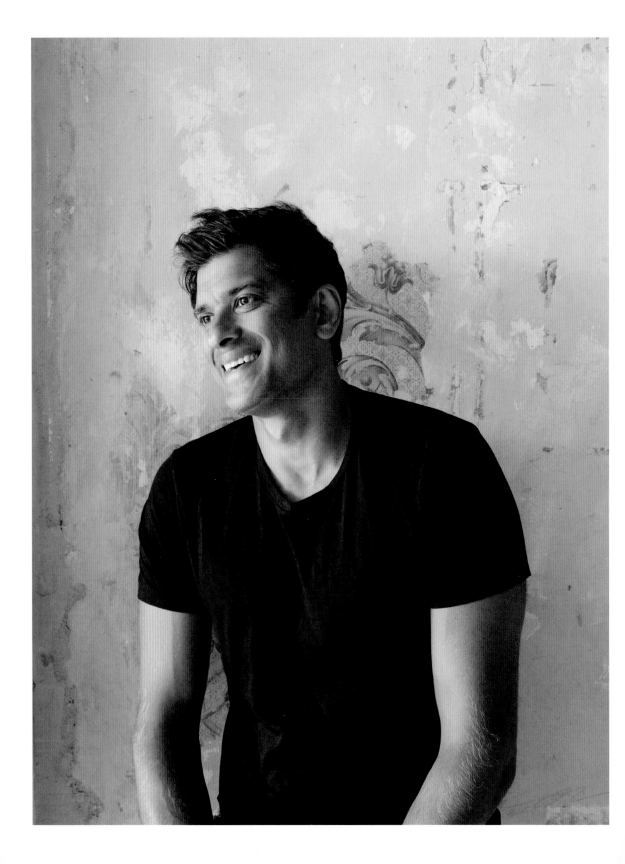

WELCOME TO SUCCESS

It never works, does it? That amazing healthy-lifestyle plan you swore you were going to stick to. That solemn resolution that you were going to exercise three times a week, eat wholesome food, and lose that excess weight that's been bothering you for years.

It starts off well enough. You begin your new regime full of energy and optimism. You smash through the first day or two, beaming with pride, convinced you'll be able to keep it up for ever. But then it gets trickier. The novelty wears off. Life gets in the way. You might last a week or two, maybe a month, perhaps even several months. But somehow, you always seem to find yourself back where you started again. So you beat yourself up. You didn't have what it takes. You didn't have the willpower. You just weren't good enough. You failed.

Wrong. The very fact that the experience I've just described is so utterly predictable should be all the proof you need that the problem isn't you. The vast majority of people who try diets and health-turnaround plans don't manage to make them stick. As a busy GP, I've seen it time and time again: smart, tough, and worried people struggling with the basics of living well and promising to do better. They would embark upon their latest health kicks full of sincere promises that this time they were going to change their habits for good, and then I'd inevitably see them in my clinic, a few months later, sad and ashamed of themselves, apologizing for their failures.

But these patients have nothing whatsoever to be ashamed of. And neither do you. The fact is, most health plans are based on the common but incorrect assumption that you can make sweeping and lasting changes to your health by relying *solely* on willpower and motivation. You've been promised you can simply decide to become a different person—a new, energetic, healthy, zingy, glowingly perfect version of you—and then become it. For the vast majority of us, this is just not true.

Most people who decide to change their lives using only willpower to get them through are pretty much doomed to fail. And the reason for that failure doesn't lie in them but in the method itself. Sure, willpower and motivation are important to get you started, but in the long term they are rarely enough. The proof is in the untold millions of sensible and determined people all over the world who've tried and tried and tried again, only to find themselves back where they started.

If this sounds like you, there's no need to despair, because in your hands you have a plan that is *finally* going to help you. This plan will not only have you feeling better within days, it will also lead to meaningful and long-lasting change. My plan is easy to follow, easy to maintain, and requires only the smallest amount of willpower.

Feel Better in 5 is a program that has been tried and tested on my patients. Busy people with busy lives, just like you. And it works so well because it has been created using the latest science on successful behavior change and because it understands that the vast majority of health problems that people suffer from today are rooted in our busy modern lifestyles.

It's revolutionary because it will lead to noticeable change without demanding that you wake up tomorrow morning and magically become a completely new you. All it asks for is five minutes of your time, three times a day, just five days a week.

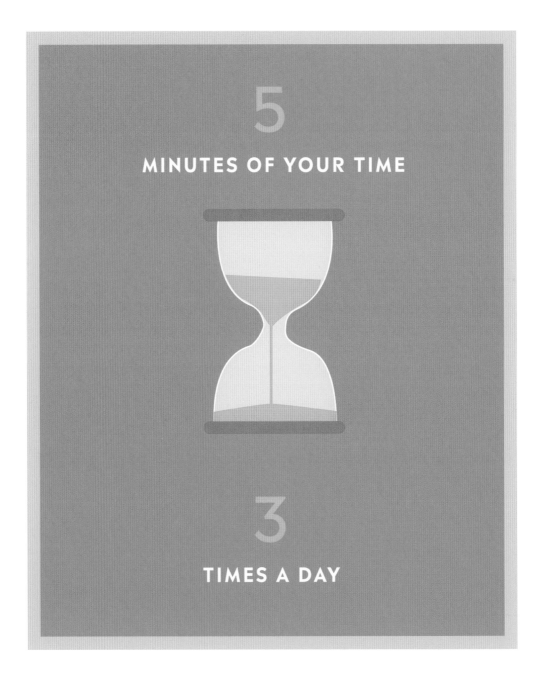

MY PLAN IS **EASY TO FOLLOW**
EASY TO MAINTAIN AND REQUIRES **ONLY**
THE SMALLEST AMOUNT OF WILLPOWER

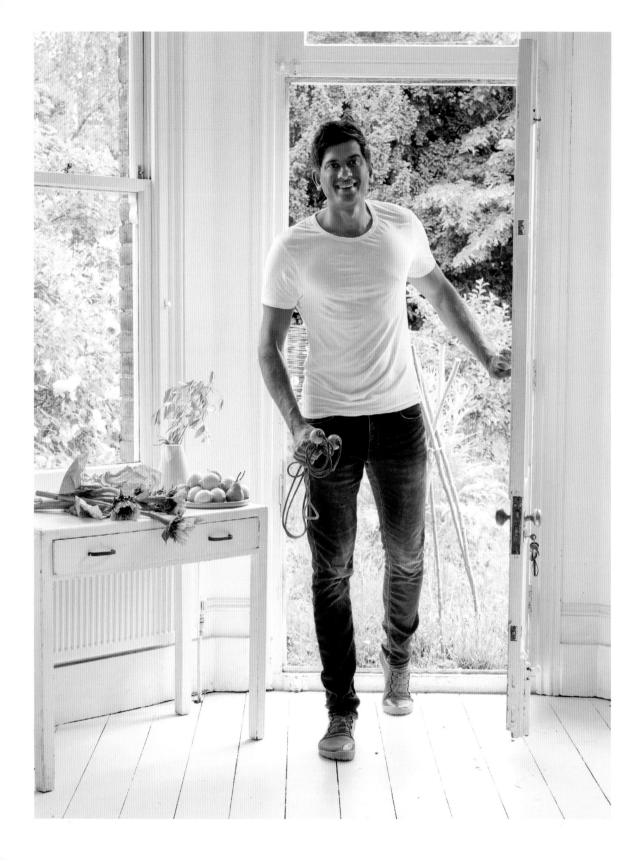

YOUR LIFE CAN BE MEDICINE

Before we rush headfirst into the details of the *Feel Better in 5* method, let's take a quick moment to understand why it is so effective. It is based on the simple fact that it is the way we choose to live, day in and day out, that mostly defines how healthy we end up being. If we consistently make good choices, we'll end up feeling well. If we repeatedly make bad ones, we'll end up struggling and getting sick. This may sound so obvious it's hardly worth saying at all. But it might surprise you to know that this is not how we currently look at health.

Imagine that you go to see your doctor, complaining of a headache. Your doctor will listen to you describe your symptoms and give you a diagnosis based upon what you've said. They may say you have a tension headache or a migraine. You'll probably then be prescribed one or more medications to help you with your pain. This is how doctors are trained. It's how I was trained, in one of the UK's top medical schools.

Of course, there's nothing necessarily wrong with giving you a pill to help reduce your pain. But I believe a much better approach would be to try to figure out the root cause of your headache. For example, it might have been triggered by not drinking enough water, excess stress, a food intolerance, too much screen time, a neck problem, or insufficient sleep. Sure, a pill might be helpful in the short term. But in the long term we should be aiming to understand *why* you got your headache in the first place.

This is the approach I've taken in *Feel Better in 5*. It recognizes that for most of us, the source of good health, as well as bad health, is our lifestyle. About 80 percent of the problems I see as a GP are not caused by a glitch in our system that simply needs fixing. Instead, they are usually a sign that something is wrong in my patient's day-to-day activities. I'm not only talking about conditions like type 2 diabetes and putting on excess weight, which many of us already recognize can be related to our lifestyles. Our collective modern ways of life also play a role in many other complaints, such as gut problems, mood issues, insomnia, low sex drive, poor concentration, hormonal complaints, and high blood pressure.

Perhaps someone is making unhealthy food choices. Perhaps it's related to stress. Perhaps there is a lack of close, nourishing relationships, or maybe there's some depression or anxiety that needs to be dealt with, or a lack of exercise or good-quality sleep. Almost certainly it's going to be more than one of these things and, more often than not, I find that it's in making small adjustments to my patients' lifestyles that the best cures can usually be found, rather than in a packet of pills.

This is the simple idea that lies at the heart of the *Feel Better in 5* method. I'm going to ask you to introduce three simple and easy practices into your daily routine, five days a week. I call these practices "health snacks." Each one of these health snacks will take no more than five minutes to complete. This is short enough for you to fit into your busy day yet long enough to ensure that you gain real benefit from doing it.

Each health snack will focus on a different aspect of your health: Mind, Body, and Heart. Often we only focus on one area when trying to improve our health, which is why the benefits are usually short-lived. For example, let's say you're trying to reduce your sugar or alcohol intake. You may be initially successful while your motivation is high. But usually, after a week or two, you will have slipped back into your usual patterns. The reason you ate sugary foods and drank too much alcohol in the first place might have been to help you manage and cope with the stress in your life. If you don't deal with the stress, you'll never change the behavior. This is why my *Feel Better in 5* method helps you tackle every aspect of your health.

By completing three short health snacks a day, you'll quickly begin to feel happier, calmer, and more energetic. You'll become physically healthier and, if you are carrying excess weight, you will start to lose it.

ONE HEALTH SNACK WILL HELP YOUR **MIND** BY REDUCING LEVELS OF STRESS AND ANXIETY.

ONE HEALTH SNACK WILL HELP YOUR **BODY** BY GETTING YOU MOVING MORE.

ONE HEALTH SNACK WILL HELP YOUR **HEART** BY STRENGTHENING YOUR ESSENTIAL CONNECTIONS.

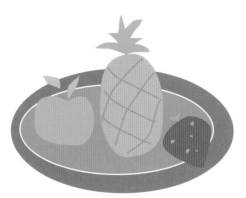

This 360-degree approach ensures that your entire system—mind, body, and heart—is being looked after.

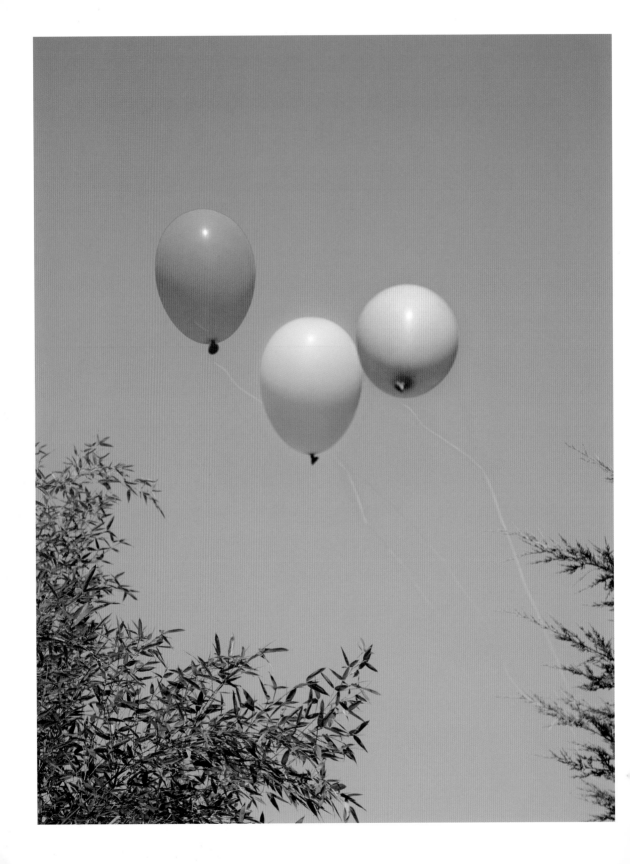

CHANGING YOUR LIFE BY CHANGING THE JOURNEY

Why don't traditional health programs work? Why do quick-fix diets fail? Why can't we simply decide to transform our lifestyles, snap our fingers, and make it happen? Because all these approaches are based on a huge but extremely common mistake. They involve thinking about health solely as a destination, about the place where we end up.

This kind of destination thinking causes even health professionals to get it wrong. Take, for example, what I've already described happening when you go to your doctor with a headache. You complain of a symptom and the doctor tries to treat it. Of course, it seems perfectly reasonable to focus on the symptom because that's the cause of the immediate distress. If someone is experiencing pain or discomfort, then that's what will naturally draw our attention. But this is the mistake. These symptoms are usually just the destination of a long journey that the patient has been on for one, five, ten, or even twenty years. While pain reduction is obviously important, the real problem is not the destination the patient has ended up at but the journey they've been on.

Take depression as another example. The symptom of low mood might be treated with an antidepressant. But low mood is just the current complaint. It's the destination where you've found yourself. Your mood problems might have their roots somewhere else that's not immediately obvious. It could be a lack of quality sleep. Poor food choices might be a significant contributory factor. It could even stem from a lack of real-life human connection or an absence of meaning and purpose.

It's precisely the same style of destination thinking that undermines our attempts at getting healthy. When we decide to turn over a new, healthy leaf, we visualize the person we dream of becoming. We fix that image in our minds and try to become that person. We see that beautiful beach body holding a perfect yoga pose or that muscleman breezing through his ten-mile run and we think, *That's who I'm going to be*. We fill ourselves with hope and motivation and aim ourselves towards that distant ideal—and then are surprised and disappointed when we lose hope and fall flat on our faces. Why do we fail? Because we're focusing on the destination rather than the journey. But that's not how we get anywhere.

A typical health journey is made up of thousands and thousands of little daily steps. It's these daily steps that the *Feel Better in 5* program targets. You're probably thinking that my promise sounds too good to be true.

Surely you can't transform your health in just fifteen minutes a day? The amazing news is you can.

If you're doubtful, think of it this way. If I were to tell you I wanted you to start smoking nonstop for five minutes a day, then eat rich chocolate biscuits for five nonstop minutes, then drink as many liters of sugary pop as you can physically swallow for five solid minutes, and that I wanted you to do this five days a week, every week, you wouldn't be at all surprised when this started changing your health. After a week or two of this madness, you'd start to feel worse. You'd have less energy. You'd start coughing. You'd start craving more and more sugary foods. The shape of your body would begin to change. After a month or two you might experience the first symptoms of more serious problems. And after a year? Two years? You may well be on the road to suffering a life-threatening disease.

Good health works in exactly the same way as bad health, yet we don't think of it in the same way. It's the journey you're taking—the small, regular, daily steps you're choosing to make—that will end up having the most dramatic long-term effects. *Feel Better in 5* is all about this journey. It's about changing your steps and taking you to an amazing, happy and healthy long life. What I've discovered in my clinic, time and time again, is that when I pay attention to my patients' journeys, it's amazing how many of their problems just vanish.

WHY DON'T YOU TAKE A FEW MINUTES TO MAP OUT YOUR OWN HEALTH JOURNEY?

ASK YOURSELF WHAT HAS BEEN GOING ON IN YOUR OWN LIFE OVER THE PAST FEW YEARS.

HOW HAVE YOU ENDED UP AT THE HEALTH DESTINATION WHERE YOU FIND YOURSELF TODAY?

WHICH PART OF YOUR JOURNEY ARE YOU HOPING TO CHANGE BY STARTING THE *FEEL BETTER IN 5* PROGRAM?

WHAT DAILY STEPS HAVE YOU BEEN TAKING OVER THE PAST FEW YEARS, AND HOW CAN YOU REPLACE THE UNHELPFUL ONES WITH NEW AND IMPROVED ONES?

WE ARE OUR HABITS

What are these tiny steps that we make every day? They're habits. And humans truly are, as it's often said, creatures of habit. Research suggests that almost half of all the activities we engage in over the course of a single day are done out of habit. Does anyone need to tell you to brush your teeth? Close your front door? Make a cup of coffee in the morning? Of course not. You carry out these little acts without thinking. But such routines can be incredibly powerful. Small, regular habits hold far more sway over our health than large and occasional activities. Allowing yourself three *Feel Better in 5* health snacks a day, and doing them regularly and consistently, is going to do you far more good than pushing yourself through a grueling gym workout once every other week.

But getting new habits to stick can be tricky. We can't simply decide to make a habit of exercising every day and expect to start doing it almost without thinking. Over the last few years I've studied and spoken with some of the world's top experts in human behavior, and one of the things they've all told me is that if we want behaviors to become habits, they have to be easy. The fact is, it's not enough to say that healthy living doesn't *have* to be hard. What these experts have taught me is that it simply *can't* be hard. If it is hard, you'll fail. That's why I've designed every health snack to be as effortless as possible—to give them the best chance of working for you.

As simple and easy as each health snack is, make no mistake: there's complex science beneath each and every one of them. These health snacks have actual biological effects on the body in the same way that prescribed medications do. They change your system. They rewire you. If you could harness the power of these snacks and put them in a pill, that pill would be hailed as a miracle and be worth billions of dollars. This is real medicine based on the real and specific problems we have today. These health snacks will help you reduce levels of persistent inflammation in your body, which is behind the development of many of today's health problems, such as type 2 diabetes, depression and heart disease. When you do some of my five-minute Body health snacks, for example, you can change the expression of your genes, wind back the aging process and increase levels of the brain hormone BDNF, which helps you make new nerve connections and may improve your mood.

But don't worry—you don't need to know anything about hormones, inflammation, or genetic expression. I've purposefully kept the science in this book as bite-sized as the health snacks. If you're interested in finding out more details about the science behind my recommendations, you can read up on it in my previous books or listen to my free weekly podcast *Feel Better, Live More*. And if you couldn't care less? That's absolutely fine. You don't have to.

All you have to do to improve your health is give me fifteen minutes a day, five days a week.

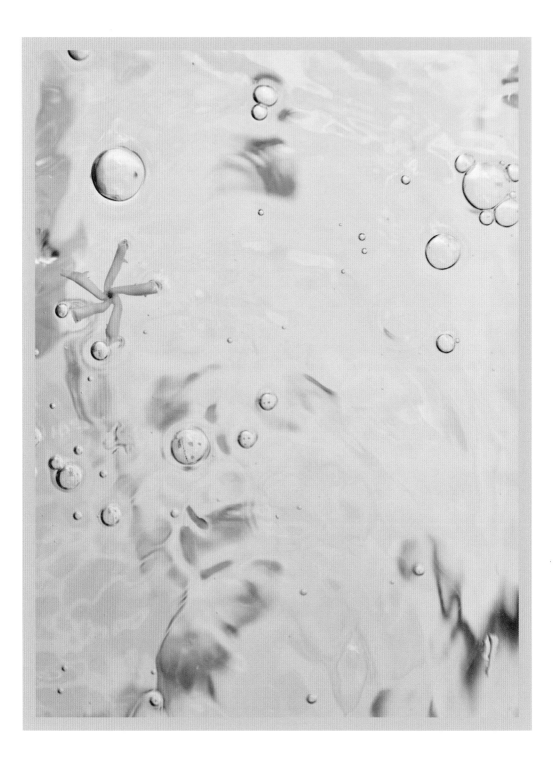

THE RIPPLE EFFECT

It was only when I started encouraging my patients to try five-minute health snacks for themselves that I really got a true sense of their power. I already knew that small, regular habits could rapidly build up and ultimately have much greater effects on health than large interventions that were less frequent and would inevitably be abandoned after a few weeks. But a second force came into play that I wasn't fully expecting. It would amplify the effects of *Feel Better in 5* to a sometimes life-changing degree. I call it the "Ripple Effect."

I see the Ripple Effect again and again. It happens when the tiny changes in routine I recommend trigger new, positive changes in other areas of my patients' lives. For example, a patient who starts doing a five-minute Body health snack will begin to feel the difference that regular exercise is making and find themselves motivated to stop eating junk food. Another who finds themselves less stressed after doing a daily Mind health snack will find that they're sleeping better, which means their performance at work improves, their self-esteem starts to rise, they feel less need for caffeine, and have more energy for exercise.

Of course, I shouldn't really have been surprised by this. I've been talking for years about the fact that our minds and bodies are all part of one connected system. Tweak one small part of our health and other pieces of it will also begin to change and improve. What this has taught me is that the lives we live work in exactly the same way as our health. We don't have a working life and a sleeping life and a gym life and a love life and a sex life and a food life and a fun life, as we often imagine. We're not compartmentalized. All these different domains are just parts of one single life. Improve one piece of it, and the benefits will spread into many different areas. It's only when you see the power of habits working in combination with the power of the Ripple Effect that you understand the true life-changing potential of the *Feel Better in 5* program.

SIX TIPS FOR MAKING CHANGES THAT STICK

All of us have made short-term changes before. But how do you get them to last for longer? Here are six of my top tips from the latest science in behavior change.

1 START EASY

It's important to kick off with snacks that last for only five minutes because the latest science of successful behavior change tells us that if we want to create new habits it's essential to start easy. One of the world's leading behavior-change scientists, the Stanford University psychologist B. J. Fogg, often tells an amazing story about how he turned the chore of flossing his teeth into a habit by starting with just one tooth. He turned it into a task that took hardly any effort. Very little willpower or motivation was required. And then what happened? After finishing one tooth, he found he just naturally wanted to do another. And then another. And then another. After a month he found that he was automatically flossing all of his teeth twice a day. It had become a new habit.

Decades of research into behavior change has found that if we want behaviors to become habitual and automatic, they should take little mental or physical effort. The easier you make a behavior, the less motivation you require to do it. This is important as motivation naturally goes up and down over time. If you've ever wondered why your smartphone is so addictive, it's because Silicon Valley uses these very same psychological techniques to keep you glued to their apps. But I want to use these powerful techniques for good—to create habits that help you rather than harm you. The *Feel Better in 5* program has been designed to give you a balance between ease and simplicity and effectiveness. Each snack should be easy enough for you to complete without much effort or cost, while being powerful enough that you should start feeling the benefits quickly.

2 CONNECT EACH SNACK TO AN EXISTING HABIT

Here's another tremendously helpful trick for turning new activities into habits. All the best researchers into behavior change recommend connecting them to

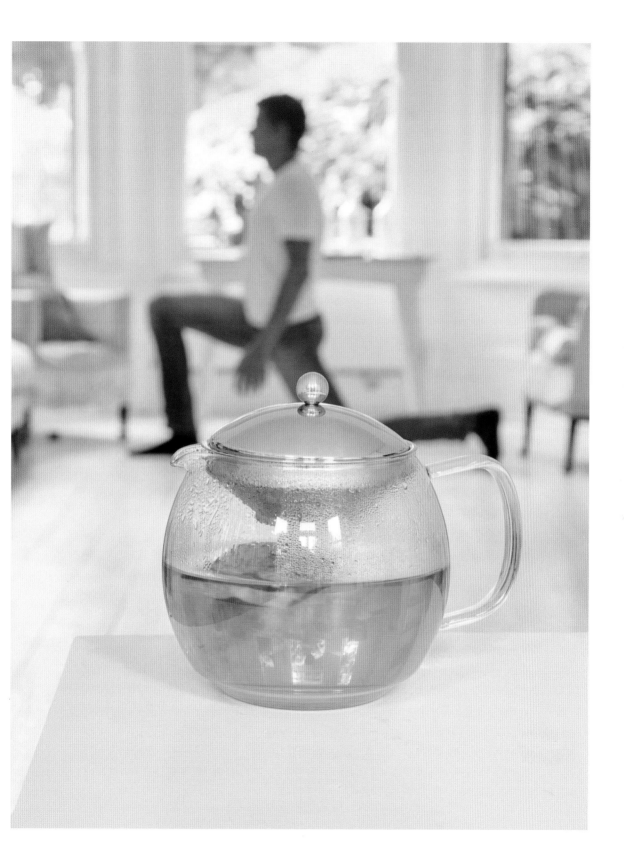

existing habits. Take Fogg and his flossing, for example. He started by giving himself a new rule: "After I brush my teeth, I will floss one tooth." He found one daily automatic behavior that was already well established—brushing his teeth—and simply hooked this new habit up to it. I'd also recommend that you do this. We're all extremely busy these days, so if you don't need to find extra time in your daily routine to fit in new activities you're much more likely to succeed.

So what are some daily routines that are already in place that you could hitch a health snack to? Most of us have a hot drink in the morning. That's a perfect place to stick on a habit. I get my own five-minute workout done when the kettle's on and my morning cup of tea is brewing. Before I've even started the day I've given myself a victory, and it feels amazing. You might also want to think about the various transition points in your day. What about when you walk into the house after work or just after you have dropped the kids off at school? Do you commute on the train? Could you get into the habit of doing a Heart health snack like writing in your gratitude journal for the first five minutes of your journey home? The important thing is that you try to stick your health snacks on to a habit that's already there. When you do this, you make it much more likely that this new behavior will become a regular part of your daily routine.

Importantly, if you try to stick your habit onto a part of your daily routine and you find it doesn't work, don't beat yourself up about it. Simply try a different slot in your day instead. Be pleased that you are learning more about what works for you and what doesn't.

3 RESPECT YOUR RHYTHM

It's also well worth thinking about whereabouts in the day you'll place each kind of snack. This is because we all have natural daily rhythms and will feel more inclined to do certain things at certain times. For example, we tend to have peak muscular strength at three or four p.m. If that sounds like you, you might want to root your daily Body health snack onto something that you already do during that period. For example, as you "transition" from the stresses of the work day to the relaxation of being at home, you could stick on a habit here. You could walk through the front door in your work clothes, change into your workout gear, and, before you do anything else (like mindlessly scroll through Instagram for twenty minutes!), you could do a five-minute yoga sequence to help you unwind both physically and mentally.

Or what about before breakfast, when your system is full of the hormone cortisol that helps you get up and attack the day? For most people, motivation is high at this time. If you do a five-minute Body health snack before your meal, your blood sugar won't rise as much. The short burst of exercise will leave your body hungry for that sugar. So you're changing the way your body processes your breakfast. In the evening, levels of the sleep hormone melatonin are usually high. Melatonin is what helps you get to sleep. You might find it helpful to work with that natural slowdown by getting into the habit of doing a thoughtful and calming Heart health snack in the evening. This will help you reframe all that negative chatter that's built up over the stresses of the day and give yourself a moment of healing, which will benefit the quality of your sleep.

The important thing is that you do what feels right for you when it feels right. *Feel Better in 5* **is a program that doesn't force you to bend your life around its demands. It bends around your life.**

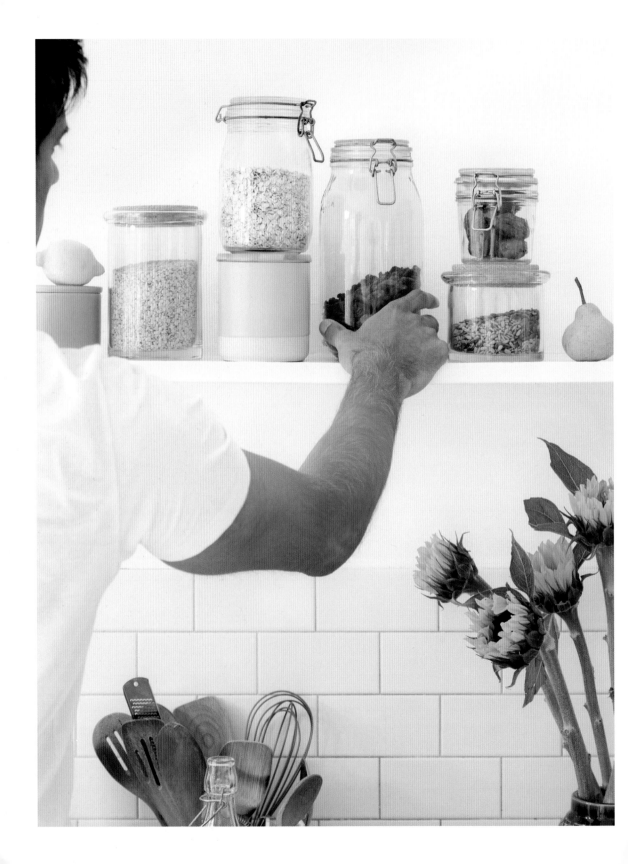

4 DESIGN YOUR ENVIRONMENT

The fact is, we humans are massively influenced by our environments. By designing your environment for success, you will go a long way to making your *Feel Better in 5* journey successful. Here are some hacks and tips you might want to consider.

IN THE KITCHEN

- Leave a step by the kitchen counter that you can use for exercise.

- Leave a dumbbell by the kettle that you can work out with whenever you're waiting for the kettle to boil.

- Go through your cupboards and remove all the sugary snacks—you'll find it very hard to resist them if they're there.

- Stock up on healthy snacks: fruits, nuts, olives, hummus, etc.

- Use your freezer as a behavior barrier. If you've had one glass of wine and don't want to be tempted to have another, put the bottle in the freezer. If you're going to be tempted to go back for second helpings of the delicious dinner you've just cooked, put the leftovers in the freezer before you sit down to eat.

- If you find yourself making unhealthy food choices in the supermarket, consider ordering your groceries online.

- Brush your teeth after you've eaten your evening meal so you're less likely to snack before bed.

 To hear more about how much our environment influences our behavior, listen to my eye-opening *Feel Better, Live More* podcast with Dan Buettner at drchatterjee.com/bluezones

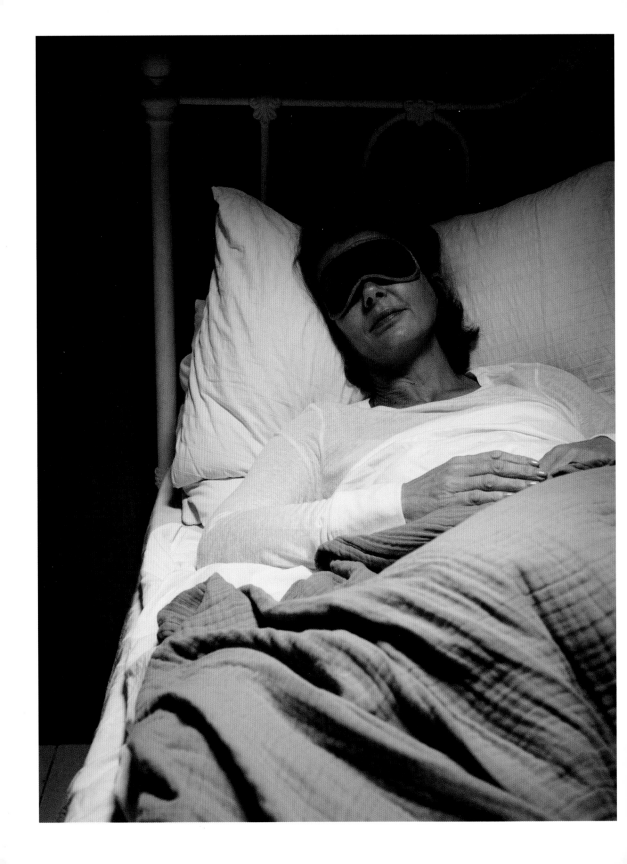

IN THE BEDROOM

- Minimize light from blinds and curtains. Consider buying blackout curtains if you can.

- Cover any LED lights from electronic gadgets. Special stickers designed for this purpose can be bought cheaply online, or you can just use some gaffer tape.

- Consider removing the television from your bedroom.

- Don't bring your phone into the bedroom. Charge it in another room.

- Consider sleeping with earplugs and an eye mask.

- Make your bed in the morning so you have an inviting and restful space to return to at the end of the day.

ON YOUR PHONE

- Change your phone to grayscale. Many of my patients report that simply removing the colors from their home screen is hugely effective in nudging them to pick it up less often.

- Leave it in another room while you are relaxing.

- Remove your social media apps so you can only access them through the browser.

- Sign out of your social media accounts and disable the auto-sign-in setting so you have to log in manually each time.

- Turn off fingerprint reader or face scanner so that you have to enter your PIN number.

5 USE POSITIVE SELF-TALK

If many of us talked to other people the way we talk to ourselves, we wouldn't be able to get through a single day without being slapped or shouted at. It's a sad fact that we're often our own most harsh and unforgiving judges. By making a few adjustments in the way we talk to ourselves, we can massively increase our sense of wellbeing and chances of success.

● When you're craving unhealthy food, the self-talk you choose can be critical. Don't say, "I don't eat chocolate bars anymore"; tell yourself, "Not now. I can have a chocolate bar over the weekend if I want one." By saying "not now," you're practicing healthy, journey-focused thinking, controlling what's happening in the moment, rather than what might happen in the future.

● When reminding yourself that you have a health snack coming up, don't tell yourself, "I have to do my Body health snack." Break the activity down into its very first easy step. Say, "I'm going to unroll my yoga mat."

● Don't use words and phrases like "should," "need," or "I have to." Instead say, "It would be great to . . . ," "I'll feel more energetic when I . . . ," "I'll feel calmer after I . . ."

● If you're the kind of person who feels guilty about taking me-time, reframe it. Say something like, "I'm going to be a better mom today if I do my five-minute health snack."

● Be your own best friend. When you have completed a health snack, don't be afraid to pat yourself on the back and feel great about your victory. You could try saying, "Yes!", "Excellent!", or "Good for me." You could even try singing a quick celebratory song in your head. **Although this may feel a bit silly at first, please don't underestimate its impact.**

Celebrating in this manner every time you complete a health snack is highly effective. In fact, the more intense the positive emotion you feel alongside your new behavior, the quicker you will turn it into an automatic habit. Just think, when you are feeling low and eat a chocolate bar, you immediately feel happy. This helps to lock in this behavior, so every time you are feeling low you have a craving to reach for that chocolate bar. We can use the same psychology to help us install healthy behaviors.

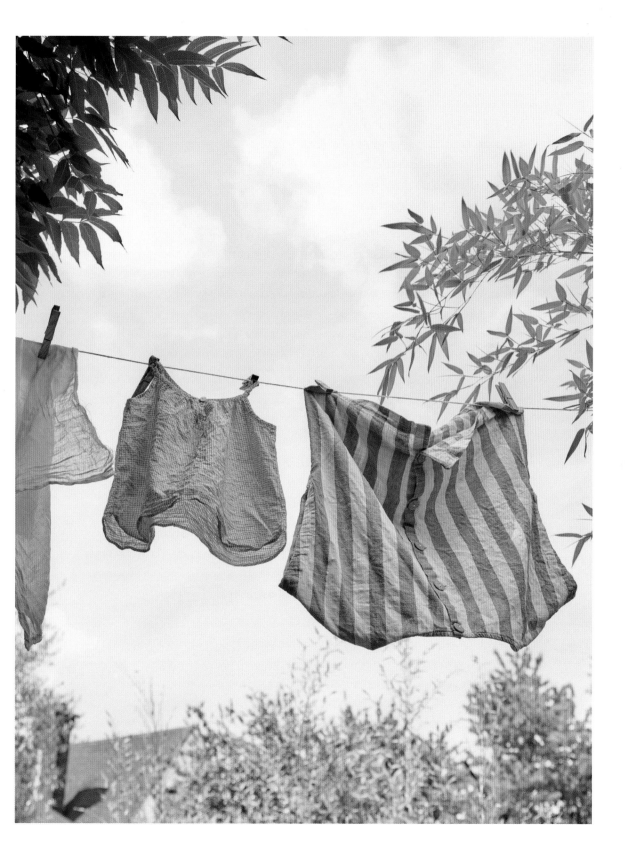

6 CELEBRATE YOUR SUCCESS

We often imagine that the right time to celebrate success is when we finally reach our distant goal. But if we only allow ourselves to feel good when we get there, we're dooming ourselves to failure. The latest science tells us that it is essential to celebrate *every* single time you make another step on your journey. Health isn't some distant goal. It's not something you become. Health is something you do. And every time you do it you're being the person you want to be.

A fantastic tip for allowing yourself to experience a little hit of pleasure every time you complete a health snack is to make it visual. Part of the problem with lifestyle choice is that you don't always see instant results. If we could actually see the damage that each double cheeseburger does to us, the cheeseburger business would collapse overnight. Likewise, if we could see the benefits that each healthy workout does to our minds and bodies, we would be doing them every day without fail.

Here's a simple trick that's worked incredibly well for a huge number of my patients. Take an old glass jar or mason jar and, every time you complete a snack, drop a single coffee bean (or any other bean!) into it. This might sound crazy, but there's just something about this action that reinforces your health habit. You can't drop the bean into the jar without feeling your victory in a really palpable way. As you see the beans collect over the weeks and months, you start to build a powerful representation of just how much all your good work is piling up.

Some people prefer a different approach. One of my patients uses a wall chart and stickers to track his workouts. Seeing all the days he's managed to get in some exercise provides him with all the motivation he needs to keep going. He has a visual record of his success and doesn't want to see his streak being broken.

At the back of this book (pages 262–63), I've created a wall chart for you to use, if you wish. Once you have ticked off your health snacks for a few days in a row, you will start to build momentum and you won't want to stop. In my experience, celebrating every single little success is just so important. We start to crave those small moments of victory. We feel bad if we miss them. When this happens to you, you'll know the program is working. You're changing your journey . . . and that's going to change everything.

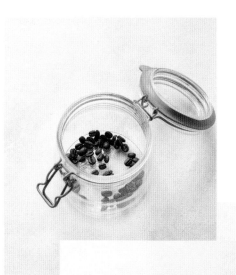

Don't miss out on the power of celebrating each health snack. It will hugely increase your chances of success!

HOW TO DO THE PLAN

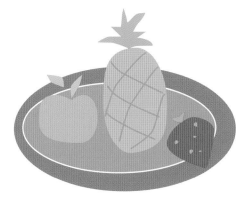

FEEL BETTER IN 5 IS A PROGRAM THAT DOESN'T FORCE YOU TO BEND YOUR LIFE AROUND ITS DEMANDS. **IT BENDS AROUND YOUR LIFE.**

It could hardly be simpler. I want you to flick through this book and choose one health snack from each of the three menus—Mind, Body, and Heart—then add them into your daily routine for five days of the week. These five days are what I call your "Feel Better Days." For some of you, they may be Monday to Friday, as these are the days when you can anchor them around the regularity of your work routine. For those with different schedules, they might be different days. Feel free to choose whichever five days you like, or do them every day of the week if you really get on a roll.

It's also up to you *when* you do your health snacks. You could do one in the morning, one at lunchtime, and one in the evening. Alternatively, you could do all three as soon as you wake up. Whatever you prefer. I have, however, suggested a time of day for some of the health snacks where I have seen them have the most impactful results.

I'd strongly encourage you to stick with the same three health snacks each day as much as you can, as this will greatly increase your chances of making each one a habit that you start to crave, just as you might crave a chocolate bar or a glass of wine. As with everything I have recommended in this book, there is no downside to doing them. None of them has harmful side effects. The worst-case scenario of doing them is you will feel slightly better than you currently do. Best-case scenario? You will change your life, for good!

KEY FOR BENEFITS

To make the health benefits of each health snack clearer, I have created a series of icons. Alongside each section in the book, you will be able to quickly identify what benefits you will receive from engaging in any particular health snack.

- Enhances focus and concentration
- Improves mood and heightens sense of calm
- Improves sleep
- Helps to reduce excess weight
- Reduces pain
- Improves energy
- Strengthens bones
- Lowers blood pressure

MIND

DOWNLOAD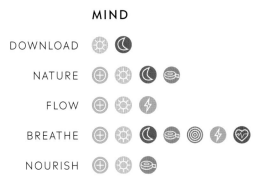

NATURE

FLOW

BREATHE

NOURISH

BODY

STRENGTH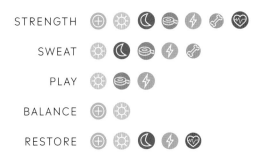

SWEAT

PLAY

BALANCE

RESTORE

HEART

CONNECT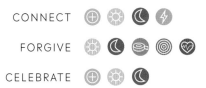

FORGIVE

CELEBRATE

HOW TO CHOOSE YOUR HEALTH SNACKS

As you read through the book you'll see there are dozens of different health snacks that you can choose from. Given that you only need to choose one from each section, the variety of choice might seem overwhelming. To make things easier, I've created a series of combinations that work particularly well for certain conditions and concerns that people regularly come to see me about as a doctor.

If you have a particular health concern you'd like to focus on—be it anxiety, depression, or high blood pressure—I've selected a series of combinations for you that you may find useful. Alternatively, if you have something that you want more of in life—such as focus, energy, or better sleep—there are plenty of options for you as well. This is a plan that is relevant for each and every single one of us, whether we feel unwell or simply want to optimize our wellbeing.

The combinations I've selected are simply the ones I've found to work well in the past. You are free to choose whichever three health snacks you want, but if you need a bit of direction, they're a useful place to start. It's very important, though, that you choose the health snacks that you really *want* to do. If I've recommended a particular heath snack that doesn't appeal, I would suggest that you don't do it. It is very hard to create new habits for things that we don't have a strong desire to do. Ultimately, doing any combination of three health snacks from this book consistently will help you improve your health and, likely, transform your life.

To see a full list of all the health snacks, please see the health snacks index on page 268.

REMEMBER, YOU **ONLY** NEED TO CHOOSE

ONE

HEALTH SNACK FROM **MIND**

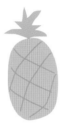

ONE

HEALTH SNACK FROM **BODY**

ONE

HEALTH SNACK FROM **HEART**

HOW TO GET LESS ...

ANGER

Feelings of hard-to-control anger can often come from feeling stressed and holding on to negative emotions. Breathing practices such as **Breath Counting** (page 96) can help you let go of pent-up emotions, while a short, intense workout that makes you sweat, such as **The Power 5** (page 136), can burn off stored-up emotional energy. **The Forgiveness Practice** (page 228) is great for releasing intense feelings of resentment that can be corrosive to mental health.

ANXIETY

When you're anxious, it can often feel like you have a million thoughts running around your head. A morning Download, such as **The 5-Step Release** (page 69), allows you to get these anxieties on paper, which can be calming. The **Simple Sweat** workout (page 143) will help you quickly burn off excess nervous energy, and a daily practice of **Reframe the Moment** (page 250) helps you to be kind to yourself, calms the mind, and takes the body out of its tense fight-or-flight state.

BACK PAIN

I know from years of agonizing experience how much back pain can get you down and affect your ability to do the things you love. While it's impossible to give a single combination that will help every sufferer, the following three health snacks often work brilliantly. **5 Minutes of Flow** (page 87) helps fully immerse the mind so attention is taken away from the soreness. The Balance workouts, like the **Desk Jockey Workout** (page 169), contain movements that help to address many of the muscular imbalances that result from our sedentary lifestyles. The **Celebrate Yourself** health snack (page 247) helps you practice self-love, which helps reduce stress levels, which in turn can play a huge role in improving back pain.

CHRONIC PAIN

Chronic pain is, sadly, extremely common and can have a devastating impact on quality of life. Painkillers usually don't fully numb the pain and can come with intolerable side effects. The **Simple Breathing** practice (page 94) will reduce your perception of pain, while the relaxing **Morning Wake-Up Flow** (page 191) can restore balance to your mind and body. The stress caused by unresolved emotions can often contribute to chronic pain and I've found that a daily practice of forgiveness, such as **The Forgiveness Affirmation** (page 231), can be tremendously helpful in easing it.

DEPRESSION

When you're feeling depressed, it can be hard to motivate yourself to do anything at all, let alone stick to a tough wellbeing regime. The beauty of *Feel Better in 5* is that each health snack takes *only* five minutes and each one will tackle a different cause of your low mood. Making a nourishing smoothie, such as **Mind the Blueberries** (page 105), feeds your brain the optimum nutrients it needs to function well. A daily practice of playful movement, such as **Dancing** (page 159), will get your body moving in an exhilarating, joyful way. Connecting with others is one of the most powerful ways of lifting your mood. This can be hard to do when you're feeling especially low, so you might want to consider starting with **Celebrate Others** (page 248), which can feel less intimidating.

EXCESS WEIGHT

If you feel you're carrying excess weight, you've probably already tried changing your diet more than once. While this is important, there are many other factors to consider when it comes to weight. Long-term stress can cause your body to hold on to excess fat. The **Simple Breathing** exercise (page 94) will help you slow down and focus on yourself, which is a great way of reducing stress levels. The five-minute Sweat workouts, such as **The Easy Kneesy** (page 146), target fat loss and have the added bonus of being really quick and lots of fun. In my clinic, I've seen that holding on to negative emotions and not feeling good enough can also contribute to excess weight gain. These issues cause long-term stress and often lead to the overconsumption of sugar and alcohol. The **Celebrate Yourself** health snack (page 247) or **The Forgiveness Practice** (page 228) can help you start to address these areas.

GUT ISSUES

About seventy-five percent of people in the US suffer from a gut-related problem each year, so pretty much all of us will encounter one at some point. While the foods we choose contribute to this, our busy and stressful lifestyles are probably an even bigger factor. **The Gut Bugs Health Snack** (page 108) will help feed your gut bugs the nutrients they love. **The Day's End Release Flow** (page 195) will provide your body with the gentle movement your gut really likes. Stress will exacerbate every single gut issue, so I strongly recommend **The Love List** (page 214), which forces you to stop and really appreciate the good that others in your life do for you. This helps to reduce the stress hormone cortisol and promotes relaxation.

HEADACHES

While headaches can have many different causes, a lot of them are caused, or worsened, by stress. **5 Minutes of Flow** (page 87) can help you focus on something enjoyable, which automatically reduces stress. The relaxing **Morning Wake-Up Flow** (page 191) will help bring harmony to your body and mind. A daily practice of reframing, such as **Reframe the Moment** (page 250), can help reframe the negatives of the day and make you feel more positive.

HIGH BLOOD PRESSURE

High blood pressure is an incredibly widespread and often very serious issue. It increases your chances of developing heart disease, strokes, and dementia. Stress is a common driver of high blood pressure and five minutes of **Simple Breathing** (page 94) will help switch the body to a calmer state. Research has shown that strength training, like **The Classic 5** workout (page 119), can be helpful in lowering blood pressure, and a forgiveness practice, such as **The Forgiveness Affirmation** (page 231) can help you let go of resentment and tension that might also be playing a large role.

STRESS

The World Health Organization says that stress is *the* health epidemic of the twenty-first century. Stress can be behind a whole variety of symptoms, including insomnia, anxiety, low libido, gut problems, poor concentration, and high blood pressure. Simply spending **5 Minutes in Nature** (page 79) will directly lower levels of the stress hormone cortisol. A daily practice of yoga, such as **The Day's End Release Flow** (page 195), is one of the best forms of movement practice for dealing with chronic stress—especially the type that's prevalent these days, which comes from feeling overloaded. Regularly doing things you love by practicing **Daily Pleasure** (page 245) will make you more resilient to life's everyday stressors.

TYPE 2 DIABETES

Of course, when it comes to type 2 diabetes, there's no substitute for changing your diet.* But there are other factors at play too, and *Feel Better in 5* can help target many of them. I'd start with having a nourishing smoothie, like **Happy Brain Smoothie** (page 106), which will help put the right nutrients into your body. A regular practice of strength training, like **The Classic 5** (page 119), is essential and helps increase your body's storage capacity for sugar. For anyone with type 2 diabetes, it's crucially important to slow down and focus on yourself, as this helps to reduce levels of the stress hormone cortisol, which if left too high for too long can increase your blood sugar and exacerbate the disease. A Celebrate health snack such as **Celebrate Yourself** (page 247) will help you do exactly this.

*For more detailed information on improving your diet, see my first book, *The 4 Pillar Plan*.

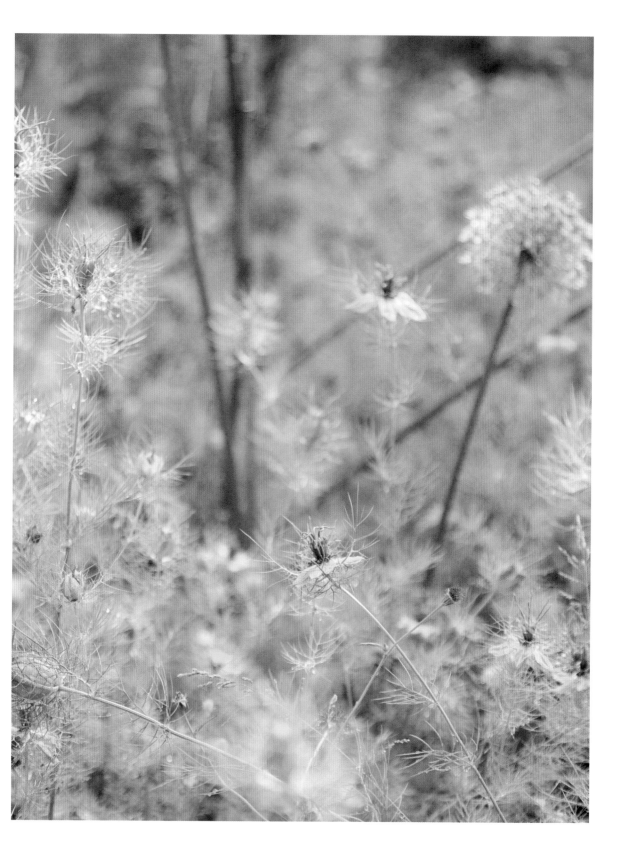

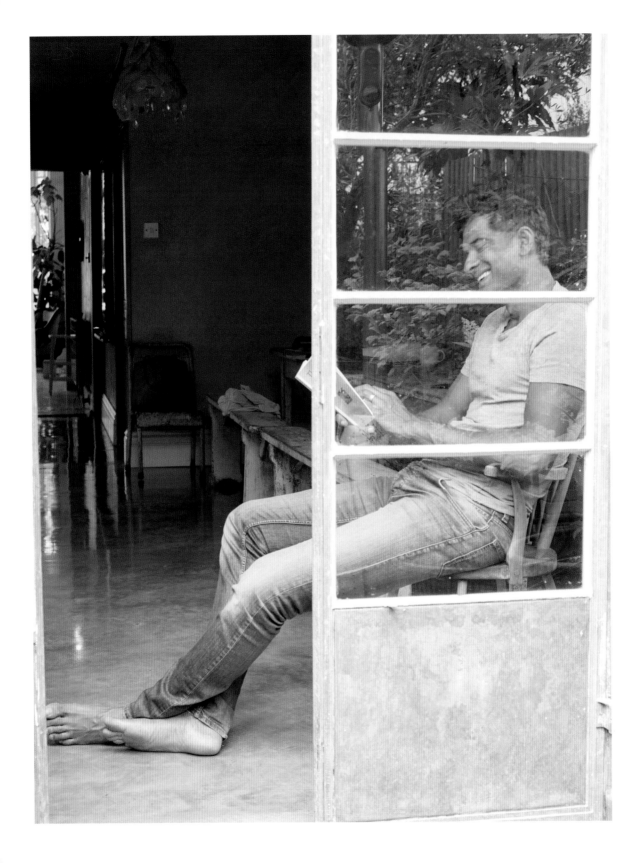

HOW TO GET MORE...

ATHLETIC PERFORMANCE

If you want to reduce your risk of injury and improve your athletic performance, a daily breathing practice can be tremendously helpful. **Breath Counting** (page 96) helps relieve stress and improves focus. Doing **The Clock Workout** (page 179) can help bulletproof your body from injury and prepare your muscles and joints for unpredictable and increased movement. The regular practice of affirmations in **Reframe the Future** (page 254) can feed your brain positive information to help prepare for your strenuous activity. Many top athletes are known to use visualization and positive self-talk to help them in the run-up to competitions. Whether it's a weekend hike, a Saturday-morning park run, or even a Tough Mudder you are preparing for, these three health snacks will help improve your performance.

BRAIN HEALTH

The good news is that there are many simple things you can do each day to improve brain health. Nourishing your body with the **Happy Brain Smoothie** (page 106) will give your brain all the nutrients it needs to thrive. **The Classic 5** Strength workout (page 119) increases levels of the hormone BDNF, which helps support new nerve connections in your brain. **Gratitude for Life** (page 239) will help you reflect on all the positives in your life, which has been shown to improve happiness and reduce depression.

CLOSER RELATIONSHIPS

Sometimes the strain in our relationships comes from not engaging in activities that make us feel alive. Accessing your flow state (page 84) regularly, with **5 Minutes of Flow** (page 87), can help address this. Five minutes of **Dancing** (page 159) can reconnect you to yourself and can be fun to do with your partner. The **Tea Ritual** (page 216), in the Connect section, can be a great way of giving your relationship a few essential minutes of focused care and attention every day.

CREATIVITY

A regular practice of **The Brain Tap** (page 66) is a great way of enhancing creativity. Often the backlog of thoughts that stays in your mind can be a block to creativity, so simply writing them out each day frees up mental capacity to be more creative. **Dancing** (page 159) is a primal form of movement that can help to unlock your creative potential. The daily practice of **Reframe the Day** (page 253) will also help get the creative juices flowing.

ENERGY

Many of us feel fatigued because we're not spending enough time doing the things we love. Regularly accessing **5 Minutes of Flow** (page 87) helps change that. Not moving enough can leave you feeling fatigued, so a quick burst of movement like **Simple Sweat** (page 143) can be incredibly helpful. When you focus your attention on celebrating all the good in your life, rather than focusing on the negative, it can be energizing. **Reframe the Day** (page 253) is perfect for this.

FAMILY HEALTH

If you want to improve the health of your whole family, the following health snacks work really well. Spending time outside together and getting **5 Minutes in Nature** (page 79) improves the way you feel instantaneously by reducing the stress hormone cortisol. A daily practice of play such as jumping rope, tag, or even having a dance together can get everyone moving and bonding. **The Gratitude Game** (page 237), which I play with my own family every night, is brilliant. It helps us focus on the positives in life and enables us to discover things about each other that would be unlikely to come up in normal conversation.

FOCUS

The modern world, and technology in particular, is constantly pulling our attention this way and that. This is affecting our ability to properly focus. Five minutes of **Breath Counting** (page 96) will increase your attention span, and five minutes of restorative yoga movements, such as **The Day's End Release Flow** (page 195), will enhance your concentration. The **Gratitude for Life** practice (page 239) improves focus by forcing you to pay attention to all the good things in your life.

HAPPINESS

If you want to feel happier, simple habits carried out each day will make a big difference. Spending **5 Minutes in Nature** (page 79) will improve psychological wellbeing, doing **The Classic 5** Strength workout (page 119) will help to improve your mood, and regularly doing **The Kindness Practice** (page 218) is one of the easiest ways to feel good about yourself.

KINDNESS TO YOURSELF

Many of us treat ourselves in ways we'd never consider inflicting on others. This can affect our mood and our sleep patterns and contribute to unhealthy lifestyle choices. While it can take time to change these patterns of behavior, these three health snacks will really help. Allowing yourself five minutes each day to focus on your breath with **Simple Breathing** (page 94) can give you some distance from everyday life, which helps you see your daily behaviors more clearly. Giving yourself five minutes each day for a restorative movement practice such as **The Day's End Release Flow** (page 195) is a great way of nurturing yourself and prioritizing relaxation. **Reframe the Moment** (page 250) is a brilliant exercise that helps you look at your life in a more understanding and compassionate way and, when practiced regularly, will result in your being much kinder to yourself in your daily life, with potentially massive benefits for health.

LONGEVITY

If staying healthy for as long as you possibly can is a priority, **5 Minutes of Flow** (page 87) will help ensure you stay mentally sharp and engaged. **The Classic 5** Strength workout (page 119) will help maintain lean muscle mass, which is one of the most important predictors of longevity. A Celebrate health snack such as

Gratitude for Life (page 239) will nudge you into focusing on life's daily small wins, and that will help your mind and body feel better.

SLEEP

Sleep deprivation is reaching epidemic levels. Most people who are struggling to sleep are doing something in their daily lifestyles that they do not realize is impacting their ability to sleep at night. Humans evolved in nature and simply exposing yourself to it, with **5 Minutes in Nature** (page 79), can help to normalize your body's daily natural rhythm, which is important for healthy sleep. A regular workout, such as **The Power 5** (page 136), helps ensure you're moving enough in the day so that you feel tired enough to sleep at night. Doing a Celebrate health snack before bed, such as **Reframe the Day** (page 253), is a fabulous way of switching your attention away from the negatives, which often keep people up at night, and redirecting it towards the positives.

WELLBEING

If none of the other categories appeal to you and you generally feel well, you might want to use *Feel Better in 5* to simply optimize your health. If this sounds like you, I'd recommend the following health snacks. A morning download such as **The Brain Tap** (page 66) is a great daily practice that helps prevent worries, anxieties, and stresses from building up and becoming harmful. **The Clock Workout** (page 179) helps ensure your muscles and joints are being moved efficiently and in different directions. This prepares them for all possible movements you may be exposed to and helps prevent injury. **Call a Friend** (page 221) will nourish your heart on a daily basis. Feeling socially connected is one of the most powerful things you can do to improve your general wellbeing.

 To hear a fascinating conversation between Mathew Walker and me about the critical importance of sleep, go to Episode 70 of my *Feel Better, Live More* podcast at drchatterjee.com/70

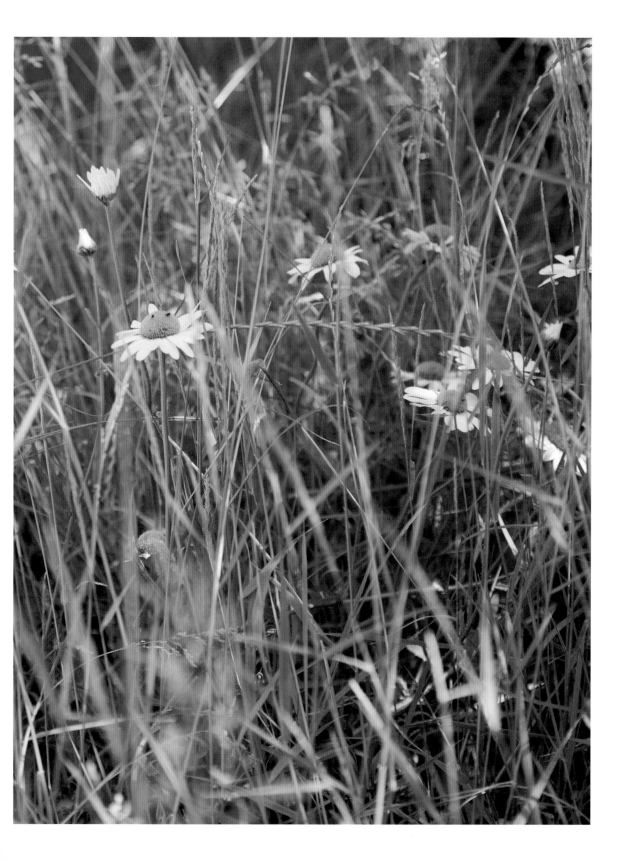

HOW TO GET LESS ...

ANGER
Breath Counting | Power 5 | Forgiveness Practice

ANXIETY
5-Step Release | Simple Sweat | Reframe the Moment

BACK PAIN
5 Minutes of Flow | Desk Jockey Workout | Celebrate Yourself

CHRONIC PAIN
Simple Breathing | Morning Wake-Up Flow | Forgiveness Affirmation

DEPRESSION
Mind the Blueberries | Dancing | Celebrate Others

EXCESS WEIGHT
Simple Breathing | Easy Kneesy | Celebrate Yourself/Forgiveness Practice

GUT ISSUES
Gut Bugs Health Snack | Day's End Release Flow | Love List

HEADACHES
5 Minutes of Flow | Morning Wake-Up Flow | Reframe the Moment

HIGH BLOOD PRESSURE
Simple Breathing | Classic 5 | Forgiveness Affirmation

STRESS
5 Minutes in Nature | Day's End Release Flow | Daily Pleasure

TYPE 2 DIABETES
Happy Brain Smoothie | Classic 5 | Celebrate Yourself

HOW TO GET MORE...

ATHLETIC PERFORMANCE
Breath Counting | Clock Workout | Reframe the Future

BRAIN HEALTH
Happy Brain Smoothie | Classic 5 | Gratitude for Life

CLOSER RELATIONSHIPS
5 Minutes of Flow | Dancing | Tea Ritual

CREATIVITY
Brain Tap | Dancing | Reframe the Day

ENERGY
5 Minutes of Flow | Simple Sweat | Reframe the Day

FAMILY HEALTH
5 Minutes in Nature | Just Play! | Gratitude Game

FOCUS
Breath Counting | Day's End Release Flow | Gratitude for Life

HAPPINESS
5 Minutes in Nature | Classic 5 | Kindness Practice

KINDNESS TO YOURSELF
Simple Breathing | Day's End Release Flow | Reframe the Moment

LONGEVITY
5 Minutes of Flow | Classic 5 | Gratitude for Life

SLEEP
5 Minutes in Nature | Power 5 | Reframe the Day

WELLBEING
Brain Tap | Clock Workout | Call a Friend

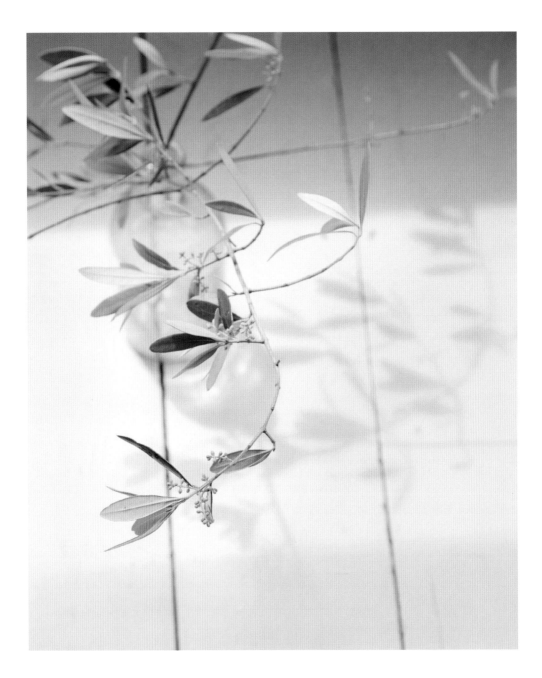

1
MIND

JUST FIVE MINUTES IN THE MORNING CAN
DRAMATICALLY IMPROVE MOOD, AND THAT'S
GOING TO INCREASE OUR CHANCES OF HAVING
A TRULY FANTASTIC DAY

MIND SNACKS MENU

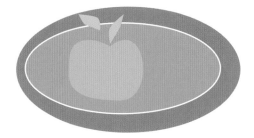

CHOOSE **ONE** HEALTH SNACK
TO **CALM YOUR MIND**

DOWNLOAD

THE BRAIN TAP | THE 5-STEP RELEASE

NATURE

5 MINUTES IN NATURE

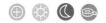

FLOW

5 MINUTES OF FLOW

BREATHE

SIMPLE BREATHING | BREATH COUNTING

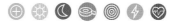

NOURISH

MIND THE BLUEBERRIES | HAPPY BRAIN SMOOTHIE

THE GUT BUGS HEALTH SNACK

MIND

Our minds are not designed for the modern world. The incredible pace of human civilization has far outrun nature's ability to update the design of our brains to help us cope with it. I'm convinced this is a big part of the reason why one in four people in the US experiences a mental health problem each year. Our minds are overloaded. We're bombarded by information and mentally drained by constant demands on our energy and time. If we want to be healthy, it's critical that we honor one of the body's most powerful yet fragile organs—the brain.

This is why, on each of your Feel Better Days, I'd like you to spend five minutes focusing on your mind. It's completely up to you to decide when to do these exercises. My recommendation, though, is that you do them in the morning. It's not uncommon for us to wake up still full of thoughts and anxieties that our subconscious minds have been churning over all night. You may have been watching the news just before bed or got into a debate online, and this can have an impact on how you feel the next morning. It can lead us to feel panicky and unsettled about the day ahead, which starts us off on a bad foot and makes it less likely that we'll make good choices during it. Just five minutes in the morning can help dramatically improve mood, and that's going to increase our chances of having a truly fantastic day.

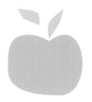

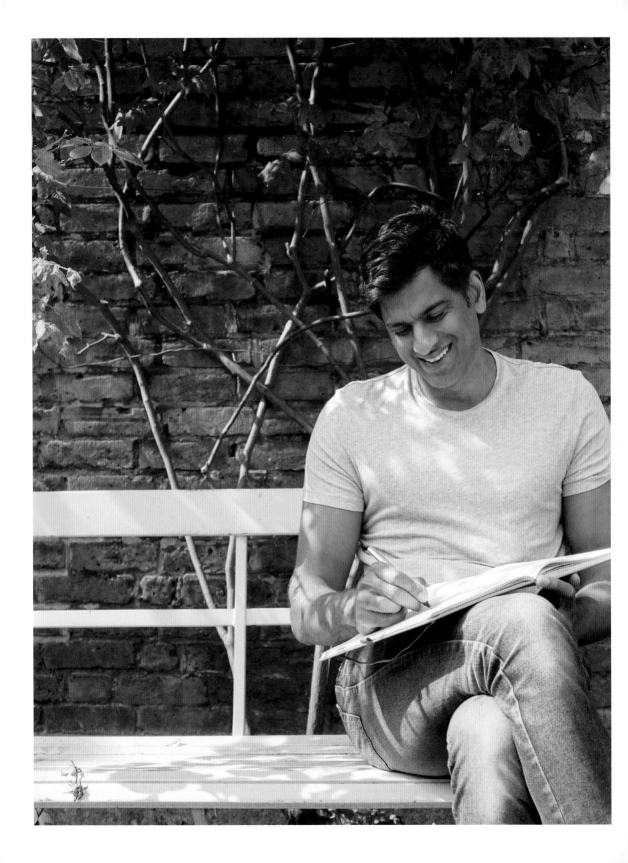

DOWNLOAD

It's a healthy part of human nature to be able to vent to those around us, but this isn't always possible with the fast-paced lives many of us now have. I like to think of downloading as my free daily session of therapy. The idea behind it is that our minds are constantly brimming with thoughts, especially first thing in the morning, when we have all the stresses and anxieties about the coming day swirling around inside us. Most of the time, we just launch into our busy schedules without doing anything to get rid of these mental worries. Time and time again, I've found that simply spending just five minutes downloading them out of your brain can have a big impact on overall health.

Some of my patients like to call this health snack a "brain dump," because you are literally dumping your thoughts out of your brain. There's something so therapeutic about seeing all that worry contained as words on a page that you can just ball up and toss in the trash. Once you start downloading regularly, you'll soon find you're living every day with a clearer and less anxious mind, and your ability to absorb the ordinary stresses of modern life will start to soar.

 You can listen to an exciting conversation between Dr. Tara Swart (neuroscientist) and me, where we discuss the power of writing down your thoughts, on my *Feel Better, Live More* podcast at drchatterjee.com/58

THE BRAIN TAP

Transfer those whirring thoughts out of your head and on to a fresh piece of paper.

I'd like you to find a quiet space, set a timer for five minutes and simply write down every thought that comes into your head as it happens. Some of my patients find this a bit difficult at first. They sit staring at the blank sheet with the timer counting down, worrying that whatever they put down is going to be wrong.

If this sounds like you, my advice is just to start. There is no "wrong" in this exercise. It's really important that you don't filter or judge yourself as you're writing. This isn't a diary, or your debut novel; it's a garbage dump. When you find your flow, you'll probably notice all sorts of craziness pouring out of yourself. It might be complete gibberish. It could be stuff that you'd hate anyone else to know. This is good. It's a sign that the process is working.

Don't be tempted to do this exercise on your phone or laptop, or tell yourself that you can just speak your thoughts out loud and process them that way. There's something about the act of physically writing it all down, with a pen or a pencil, that allows you to work through it all in a way that's incredibly powerful.

Some people find it useful to buy a journal, as this can help make your decision to create a regular practice of downloading feel committed and real. If you do decide to get a journal, treat yourself to the nicest one your budget can stretch to. Choose a color that you love and a quality of paper that feels just right. Take pride in it. Treasure it.

Of course, some of my other patients are worried about prying eyes. They'd be mortified if anyone else read their innermost thoughts, anxieties, and desires. Some of these patients lock their journal away or simply do their download each day on a fresh sheet of paper, which they then recycle or perhaps burn. They tell me there can be something profoundly symbolic about setting fire to all that toxic brain rubbish.

Note: Of course, if you do choose to burn your notes, make sure you do it somewhere safe!

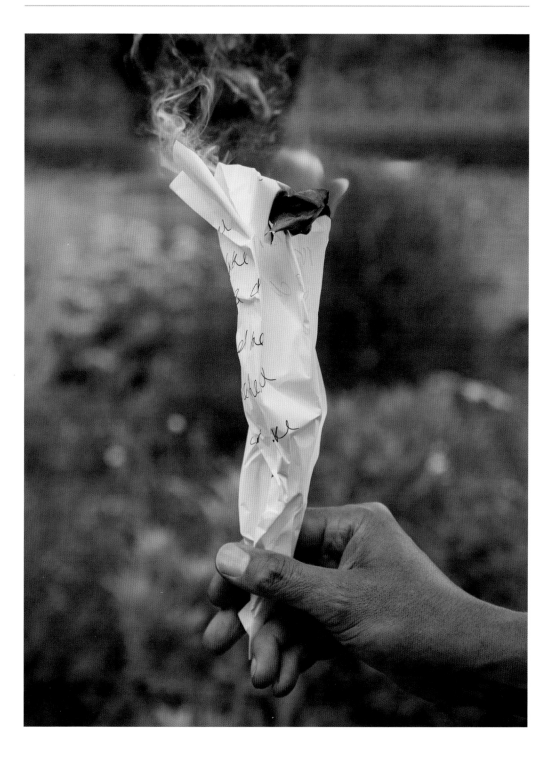

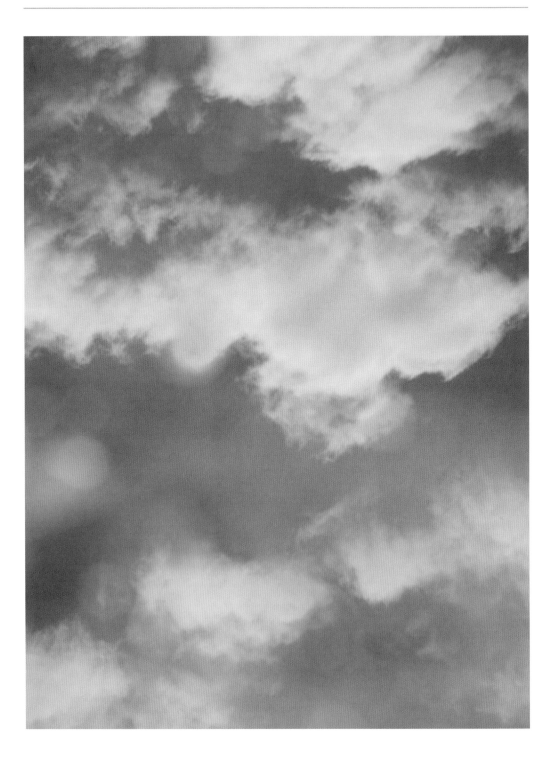

THE 5-STEP RELEASE

Set yourself up for a calm day by working through these simple steps.

Some people prefer to do their downloading with a bit more structure. If this sounds like you, try to download by addressing the following five points on a blank sheet of paper.

1 One thing I'm anxious about today
Perhaps think about the issue that's most dominant in the swirl of thoughts that's going around in your head. You might also think about focusing on something that's going to happen in the near future that's bothering you.

2 One practical thing I can do to prevent or prepare for it
Not only is it usually a good idea to be proactive in dealing with our day-to-day anxieties, the act of doing something practical can in itself help make us feel better. Do you need to make sure you've worked out your route to a meeting in advance so you're not late? Do you need to prepare three points you absolutely must get across in a difficult conversation you're going to have?

3 One reason it's *probably* not going to be as bad as I fear
It's very common for us to catastrophize about things. Our minds naturally try to prepare themselves for the worst-case scenario and we can easily start to believe that things are worse than they actually are. That difficult conversation is probably not going to end up with your being fired or your child running away. Even if you are a bit late for the meeting, nobody will really hold it against you. Try to foster a more realistic view of your problem by refusing to accept the worst-case scenario that your mind is trying to focus on.

4 One reason I know I can handle it
The chances are that, no matter what it is that's concerning you, you've been through much worse before—and survived! Try to gain perspective by remembering how you tackled a similar event (or a harder one!) and got through it.

5 One upside of the situation
Things are very rarely entirely bad. Most dark clouds really do have a silver lining. What's one upside of the problem that's worrying you?

CASE STUDY

A couple years ago a young nurse named Merope came to my clinic, complaining that she'd started having anxiety attacks at work. Seemingly out of the blue, her breathing would become rapid and she'd feel a tingling sensation in her fingers. As well as being frightening and embarrassing, these attacks began drawing some negative attention at work. The last straw came when she was trying to take blood from a patient and she started shaking, needle in hand. The patient filed a complaint. It was after this that she made an appointment with me.

I tried to understand a bit more about what was going on in Merope's life. She'd been struggling to sleep and that had led her to start drinking as many as seven cups of coffee throughout the day. I told her how much of an impact that was having on her body and asked her to limit herself to two cups each morning. I was hoping that this would allow her to have more and better-quality sleep.

But a couple of weeks later she was back in that same seat in front of me. She still wasn't sleeping. "I'm just lying in bed most of the night with my thoughts going 'round. I don't get to sleep until after three. I'm mostly thinking about all the things I haven't managed to get done at work that day, all the things I'm worried I might've got wrong, and everything I've got to do the next day."

I asked her if she had anyone in her life that she could off-load to and talk about her worries with, but she told me that, because of her work's erratic hours, she didn't see many people socially.

I suggested that Merope start each morning doing a download exercise. I asked her to write down all the thoughts that were going around her head on to a piece of paper until five minutes were up. I told her not to worry about what she was writing or about spelling and grammar. I explained that this was a way to transfer all her anxieties out of her mind and on to the page in front of her.

At first, she found the process a little odd. But when she lost a bit of that initial self-consciousness, you couldn't stop her. She began starting her day with a clearer, calmer head, and the benefits of that calmness fed forward into the whole of the rest of the day, right up to the moment she put her head on the pillow. The knowledge that she was going to download the stresses of the day when she got up allowed her to leave them alone at nighttime. She began sleeping better. Within a couple months, the frequency of her attacks had reduced by around 70 percent, and those she did have were less severe and more manageable.

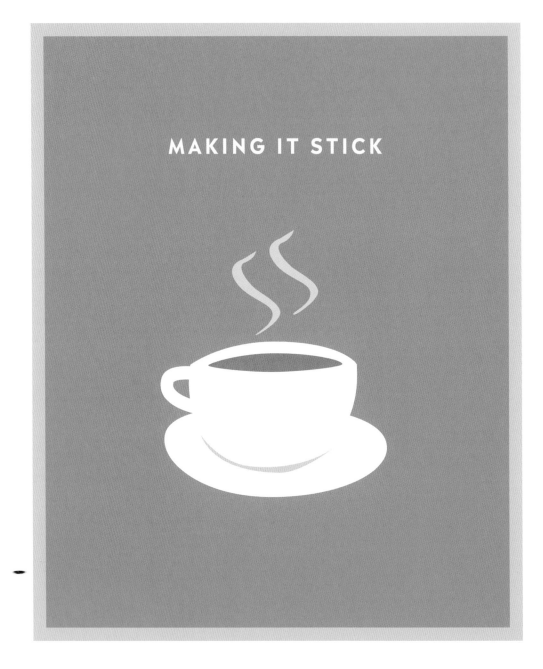

MAKING IT STICK

I recommend that you do your Download health snack first thing in the morning. This is a great habit to help launch you into your day with a calm and clear mind.

If you choose to do it just after waking, you might find it useful to put a piece of paper or your download journal next to your bed with a pen. This will act as a visual trigger that will prompt you to do your health snack.

If the first thing you do in the morning is go into the kitchen to make yourself coffee, put your journal and pen next to the coffee maker the night before. You could then take yourself to a quiet space and do your morning download while drinking your morning coffee.

If you commute to work, you might want to keep your download journal in your workbag. As soon as you're settled into your seat on the train or bus, you can start writing.

Don't forget, it's really important that you try to celebrate every time you do your health snack. Pop a sticker on your wall chart or put a bean in your jar and say something positive to yourself like, "Yes!" or "I did it!" once you are done.

NATURE

As wonderfully thrilling as cities can be, and for all the fun that can be found in your local town center, urban life can be draining. The typical modern street is a landscape that absolutely bristles with stress. Traffic, signs, ads, shops, dogs, joggers, commuters, kids, smells, honking horns, and wailing sirens—they're all signals that the brain has to work hard to process and understand as it tries to keep us alert and safe.

Compare how you feel after an hour at the shops to how you feel after an hour at the beach or in the countryside. Nature is tremendous medicine for the anxious mind. We know this intuitively, but we also know it from scientific research. Research has found that the more urban our environment, the worse our health becomes. Being out in nature has been shown to improve our mental health and our psychological wellbeing and reduce our stress levels.

We're hardwired to thrive in natural environments. We're not supposed to be boxed into airless rooms, glued to television screens, crouched over phones, or dodging traffic in polluted concrete mazes. We evolved in nature, surrounded by greenery, bathed in sky, and breathing in the healing smells of plants and trees.

 Listen to more on the benefits of nature in my conversation with Kilian Jornet on my *Feel Better, Live More* podcast at drchatterjee.com/66

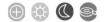

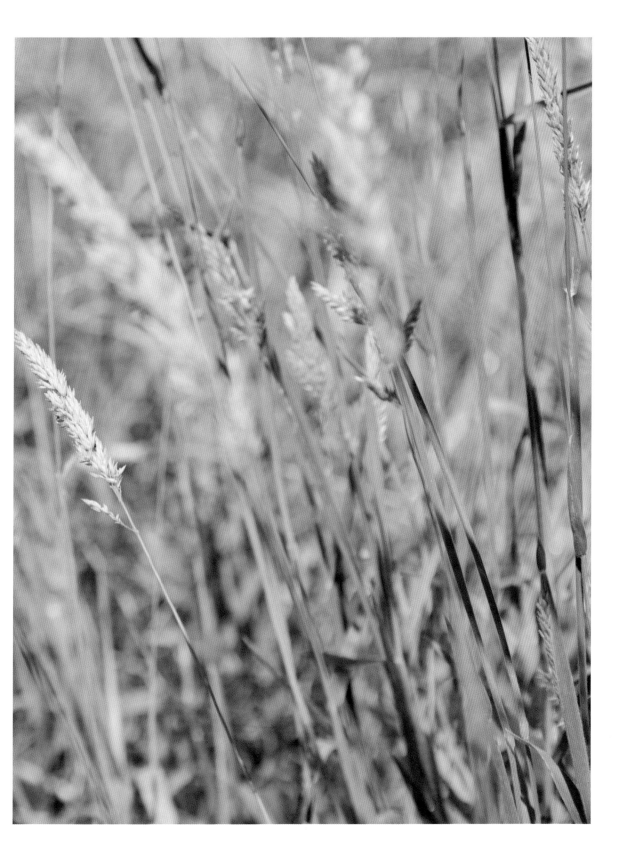

BENEFITS OF NATURE

Having more green space (parks, trees, forests, gardens, and fields) in your local environment is linked with better overall health.

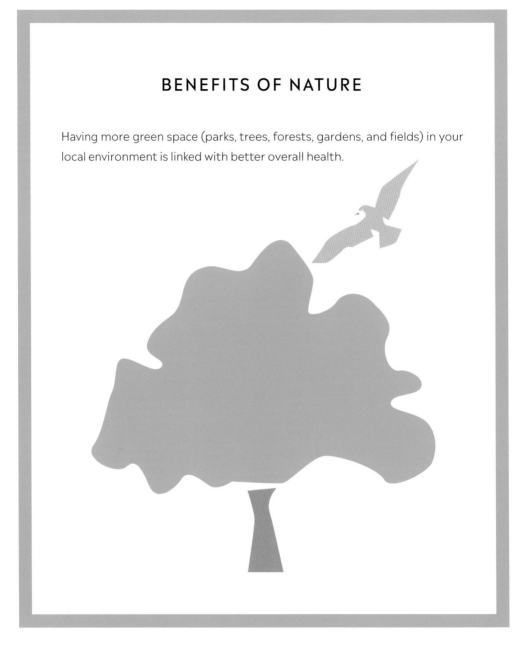

LOWERS STRESS LEVELS

Simply being in nature lowers levels of the stress hormone cortisol.

LESSENS DEPRESSION

Studies have shown that being in nature can reduce symptoms of depression.

IMPROVES MENTAL FOCUS

Spending time in nature can help increase attention span and focus.

BOOSTS THE IMMUNE SYSTEM

Trees emit certain chemicals that have been shown to have a positive effect on our immune systems.

INCREASES ENDURANCE

If we exercise in nature, rather than in a gym, we tend to exercise for longer.

REDUCES TIREDNESS

One study found that people who exercise in the outdoors on a regular basis have higher levels of a hormone called serotonin, which can help reduce tiredness and keep us in a happier mood.

REDUCES CHANCE OF DISEASE

Data from over 290 million people across twenty countries found that spending time in nature, or living near to it, can help reduce type 2 diabetes, cardiovascular disease, and high blood pressure, as well as improve sleep.

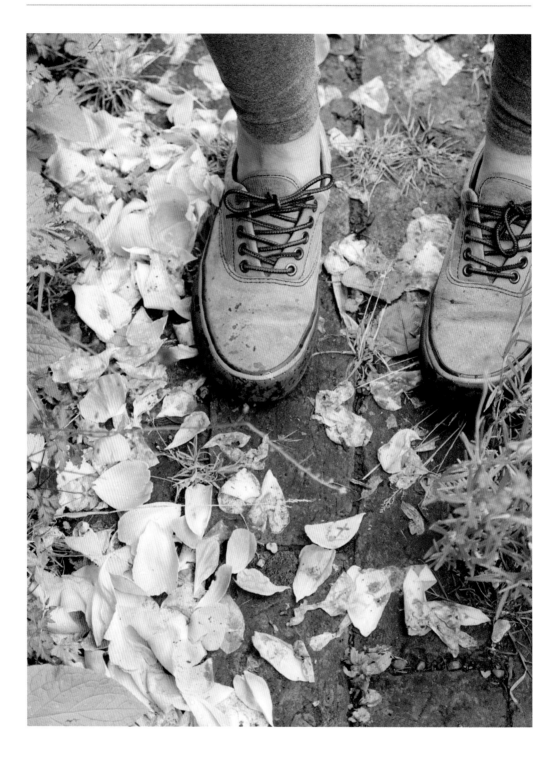

5 MINUTES IN NATURE

Spend five minutes each day enjoying nature, whether through sight, sound, or smell.

The wonderful thing about nature is that it's not only free, it's also readily accessible to many of us. If you have a yard, I'd like you to go outside for five minutes, stare at the trees, listen to the birds, watch the branches move in the wind. Really focus on your surroundings and luxuriate in the experience.

This is another health snack that's fantastic to do in the morning, as exposing ourselves to natural daylight at this time can be extremely effective in getting our natural daily rhythms in sync. It can help wake us up and, hours later, help us to sleep better.

If you wish to enhance this even further, you could go outside on to the grass with bare feet. More and more science is suggesting positive health benefits from having this direct contact with nature, but from personal experience the best reason to do this is because it feels fantastic. It wakes up the senses and is a fabulous way to start the day. This is something I try to do most mornings, even in the winter.

You can even access nature while doing something else. For example, you could have your morning cup of coffee with your window open and listen to the birds singing. Alternatively, you could drink it next to the window and meditate on the branches blowing in the wind. Or you could have your morning cup in the backyard. When I made this suggestion in my first book, *The 4 Pillar Plan*, it proved wildly popular with my readers.

There are many other ways to get creative and be in nature. For example, you could go outside and take a photo of nature each day. Perhaps you could spend a few minutes looking for the perfect frame, take some photos, and then spend the remainder of the five minutes looking through the photos and trying to choose the best one.

Alternatively, you could draw a picture while outside in nature or go outside to water and check in on your plants each day, taking the time to really notice how they have changed since the day before.

If you don't have a yard, or a nearby public green space, the sounds of nature can be of benefit. There are countless services available for free on YouTube or on streaming services such as Spotify that play the sound of waves crashing or birds singing. Get your earphones on, put your phone down, and lie in a quiet space with your eyes closed. Breathe deeply and regularly. Once again, the important thing is try to lose yourself in the experience. You can add to this health snack by introducing the smells of nature to your listening session, either by buying essential oils or lighting candles.

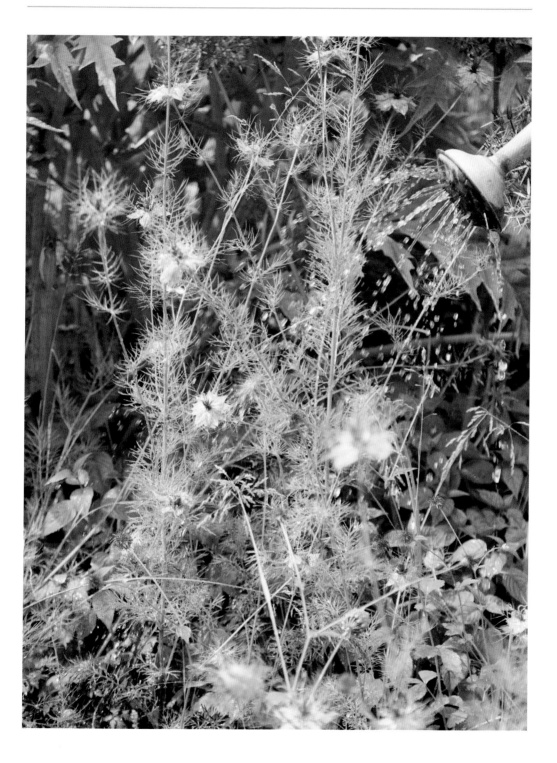

CASE STUDY

A lot of my patients intuitively understand that being in nature is good for them. But others, especially the younger ones, sometimes struggle with the idea. Twenty-six-year-old Neil, a tech worker on a tight salary living in a shared apartment in a busy town center, associated parks and open spaces with dog-walkers and sandwich-eating retirees. The only time he spent outside was walking to and from bus stops on his daily commute, and cycling along busy streets to the shops and back.

He came to my clinic complaining of insomnia and wanted the quick fix. But before I would even consider prescribing sleeping pills, I wanted to see if we could make any lifestyle tweaks that could solve his problem. I asked him what he did as soon as he woke up.

"Look at my phone," he said. He told me that he usually went straight on to social media, checked emails, or watched YouTube. I suggested that he try avoiding his phone in the morning by leaving it to charge in another room at night and to see if he could give himself a tech-free half-hour first thing every morning.

He was fairly skeptical about my recommendation and asked if there was anything else I could suggest. It seemed obvious there was no way I was going to convince Neil to part with his phone, even for a short period of time, and I'm well aware that the most successful health interventions are the ones that fit around the lives of the people I'm treating, rather than the other way around. I suggested that for the first five minutes of every day, before looking at anything else, Neil should go on to YouTube or Spotify and listen to a recording of waves crashing for five full minutes.

Neil took to the idea immediately. The first day he tried it he felt much more energized. After a few days he started doing it while looking out of the window at the trees outside. When the weather warmed up he opened the window and enjoyed the feeling of the wind on his face. It made him feel grounded and more relaxed.

"I'm able to concentrate more in the morning," he said. "I'm not jumping around trying to focus on a hundred things at once. I'm also making fewer of those little mistakes I make when I'm stressed, like losing my keys or knocking my coffee over. I've even started going outside at lunchtime for a bit of fresh air!"

It didn't take long for the Ripple Effect (page 25) to kick in. One small change quickly led to many others. A few weeks later Neil reported that his insomnia had gone, all without the help of any medication. It started with just five minutes of focus in the morning.

FLOW

Mindfulness encourages us to be "in the moment" and comes out of Eastern concepts around Buddhism and meditation. As I've watched its huge rise in popularity I've realized two important things. First of all, we're becoming more and more stressed in our everyday lives and are crying out for ways to quiet down our noisy minds. Second, we're looking for solutions that are simpler than traditional meditation, which has a reputation for being pretty tough to master.

The good news is that we can get many of the benefits of mindfulness and meditation much more easily than you might imagine. In fact, even if you've never consciously practiced mindfulness in your life, you've definitely been in plenty of mindful states and reaped the benefits. When was the last time you were so absorbed in a pleasurable task that time seemed to just disappear? Perhaps you were cooking a fun dish or painting a picture or reading a book, or were lost in a crossword or Sudoku puzzle. What happened in your mind? All the noise and stress that was running around inside it vanished, as if by magic. You weren't fixated on the past. You weren't worrying about the future. You were present in the moment. There was only you and your task.

Psychologists call this state of mind "flow." We have a natural capacity for flow states, but we seem to find them harder to access as we get older. As children, we spend much of our time absorbed in play. When my own son is playing Lego or my daughter is painting a picture, they sometimes become so lost in what they're doing that they can't hear me talking to them. But when we grow up, there's precious little time for these lovely, restorative moments of flow.

 To hear an exciting conversation about the importance of flow, check out my *Feel Better, Live More* podcast episode with James Wallman at drchatterjee.com/64

84

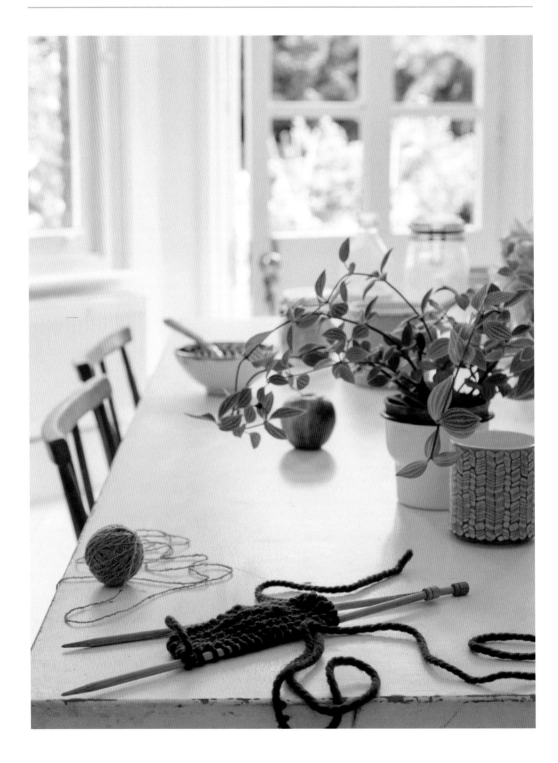

5 MINUTES OF FLOW

Devote just five minutes a day to access your flow state.

Before you start, take three deep breaths to help you relax and calm your mind. Think about what you're about to do and what you would like to achieve by doing it.

There are all kinds of activities that'll help shift you into flow. They tend to be activities that you enjoy doing. It also needs to be something that you can fully direct your attention towards, so the task needs be hard enough that you have to concentrate but not so challenging that you feel like giving up. Everyone will have a different form of activity they feel naturally drawn to. Here are a few ideas that have been especially popular with my patients.

Painting
If you like to paint, keep your brushes visible in your home and close to hand. Just get going on a project for five minutes and allow yourself to look forward to continuing on your next Feel Better Day.

Drawing
Drawing might be a little easier to get going than painting, as there is less set-up involved. Simply open up a pad, imagine what you want to draw, and do it. It is amazing how many times our children do just this. My daughter will often ask me, "Daddy, what shall I draw today?" As soon as I give her an answer, she happily opens up her book and is fully immersed in drawing. It works just as well for adults too! If you haven't finished your drawing at the end of your five minutes, carry on, if you have the time, or continue where you left off on your next Feel Better Day.

Knitting
Some of my patients love to knit. One of them, sixty-four-year-old Sheila, was suffering from anxiety. She lived by herself and would spend all day worrying about many different scenarios. She used to knit when she was younger but had not done it in years. I recommended that she dig out her knitting needles and restart for five minutes every day, to help focus her mind. Within days, she was feeling calmer, more relaxed, and happier.

Reading

If you're the kind of person who can be easily transported into the world of a book, you might be more used to reading in the evening. But many of my patients find that getting into the practice of reading in the morning can be calming. Consider reading something uplifting and motivating that puts you in a positive frame of mind to start the day.

Adult coloring books

When you're trying to color, it's almost impossible to be doing anything else but focusing on the page in front of you. Adult coloring books are one of the easiest and most enjoyable ways to practice mindfulness and access flow.

Listening to music

Listening to music can be a great way of practicing mindfulness, but only if you're fully immersed in it. It's no good scrolling through your social media feed and emails at the same time. Choose a piece of music that makes you feel good and lifts your mood. Put on your headphones. Intently follow the drumbeat or the bass line or listen carefully to the meaning behind the lyrics.

Playing music

Do you play an instrument, or did you use to? If you did, brilliant. If you didn't, it's still brilliant. You don't have to be an expert at your instrument. You're not playing for anyone else. The only thing that's important is that you're able to get lost in what you're doing. Even five minutes of playing can do wonders for your mind. One of my patients accesses flow by playing the piano. Her son takes piano lessons and when he goes to bed in the evening she looks at his piano books and tries to play the songs he's currently learning. As she becomes fully engrossed in reading the music and trying to coordinate her right and left hands, it completely switches off her mind. Afterwards, she reports feeling significantly happier and less anxious.

Jigsaw puzzles

Trying to complete a jigsaw puzzle can be a brilliant way of achieving flow state. I often do this with my children's puzzles. If this appeals to you, you can buy a variety of different jigsaw puzzles to suit your ability level. Remember, the point is simply to immerse yourself fully for five minutes.

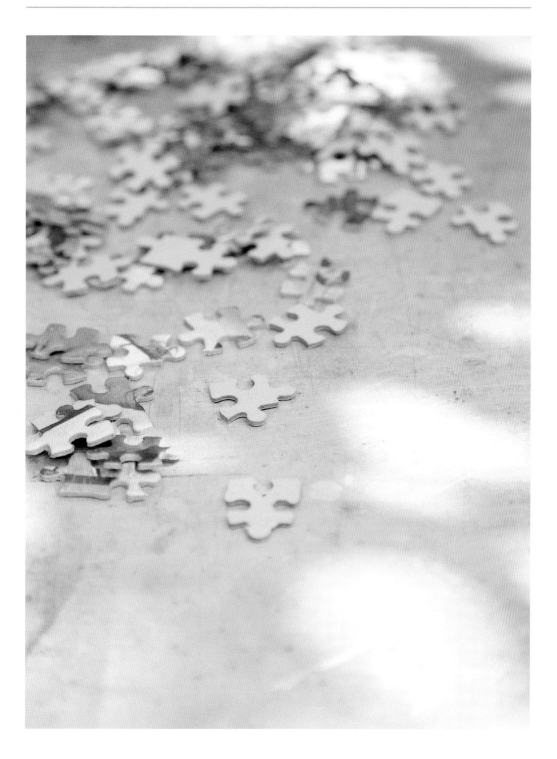

CASE STUDY

Colette was once a high-flying lawyer but had given up her career to raise her three daughters, aged between nine and fourteen. Her husband was also a lawyer and worked long hours. Like most busy parents, Colette didn't have much time for herself and seemed to be constantly busy picking her children up from school and ferrying them between clubs and play dates. When she came in to see me, Colette had been suffering from headaches across the front of her forehead for four months. She'd been taking over-the-counter medication, which was dealing with the symptoms, but she quite rightly started to worry about her reliance on them. But when she didn't take the pills she sometimes felt so poorly she became worried about her driving, which had a subsequent effect on her ability to meet the needs of her kids.

She told me that she'd wake up feeling exhausted and usually press snooze a few times. She'd then be running late, rushing around, trying to get the kids ready, and getting breakfast on the go. Her husband would leave the house at six a.m. Usually, before the end of breakfast, her headache would begin.

I asked her if she had ever tried doing any relaxation exercises. She rolled her eyes at me and said, "Meditation and mindfulness? Not for me. Sorry, Dr. Chatterjee, I know you mean well. But they're not my cup of tea. They usually leave me more irritated than when I started because I just don't feel like I'm achieving anything when I try them."

I have many patients like Colette. She was something of a perfectionist and what people used to call a Type A personality. She was all about no-nonsense forward motion, and felt in control only when she believed she was getting things done and getting them done well.

I tailored my advice to suit Colette's personality. I suggested that she buy herself an adult coloring book. Although she was initially skeptical, I managed to persuade her to give it a go. I asked her to set her alarm a little earlier, go downstairs while her kids were still sleeping, put on the kettle to boil as usual, and then, once she had made her cup of tea, sit down and color for just five minutes. I asked her to commit to this five days a week for the next two weeks.

I could tell there wasn't a single atom in Colette's being that believed this was going to work. When she came in a couple of weeks later, she told me she hadn't managed to keep it up. She either forgot altogether or decided, in the moment, that she had more important things to do with her five minutes than sitting down with her colored pencils. But I wasn't going to give up that easily. I told her a little bit about the science of behavior change and how, ideally, you need to change your environment to make the new behavior you are trying to engage in as easy as possible. I asked her to leave her coloring book next to her kettle with her pen and pick it up as the kettle was coming to the boil. And that's what did it. Keeping the book there hooked the action of coloring into her existing habit of making tea. To her surprise, she began looking forward to doing it every morning. They were "precious" minutes, she told me a few weeks later, in which she forgot everything else that was going on and got lost in a simple creative pleasure. She'd achieved flow, on a daily basis, and after four weeks her headaches had almost completely disappeared.

BREATHE

Many of my patients are reluctant to try meditation because it can sound difficult and perhaps even strange. They often assume you have to kneel down in uncomfortable positions, listen out for tinging bells, and chant, all while struggling to clear your mind so it's completely empty. Who's got time for all that?

Of course, these popular ideas about meditation are often wrong and millions of people find the practice extremely helpful. But I also understand people's reluctance in the face of the harsh realities of modern life. As much as I'd like to, I almost never find half an hour every day to meditate. I know most of my patients are in a similar situation.

Luckily, I don't have to give up half an hour a day to get many of the benefits of meditation, and neither do you. At the heart of it is simply breathing. I've honed a selection of breathing exercises that are incredibly easy and quick, and they can deliver a lot of the benefits of meditation, such as stress reduction, pain relief, increased focus, and better sleep quality. They can be done almost anywhere, as frequently as you like—unlike other powerful medicines, you can't really overdose on breathing. But I'd like you to start by finding a place in your daily schedule in which you can insert one regular breath-based health snack on each of your Feel Better Days.

One of the things many people don't realize is that, as well as keeping us alive, breathing acts as information to the brain. When we're anxious or angry, our breathing becomes rapid and shallow. The brain notices this and reads it as a signal that the world around us has become stressful and unsafe. But the opposite is also true. If we breathe in a slow and relaxed way, we send a signal to our brains that the world around us is safe and calm.

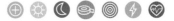

It's important to remember that, despite what you may have heard, the goal of these exercises is not to have a clear mind. Thoughts are part and parcel of normal life. The idea is to focus on your breath and catch your thoughts when they occur to you. Notice that your mind has wandered. Then, without any judgment, return your attention to the breath.

Over time, you'll come to realize that, no matter how overwhelming your thoughts and feelings seem, you don't have to let them control you. You're separate from them. You'll become better at observing them and allowing your negative thoughts to just trail off like steam from a kettle.

SIMPLE BREATHING

Spend five minutes simply focusing on your breath.

This simple health snack is perfect for everyone, no matter how experienced you are at mindfulness or breathing exercises. It's also a great place to start if you're a beginner.

It's particularly good when you're feeling anxious or are in physical pain. If your mobility is limited and you struggle to get on the floor or up again, you can easily do this sitting in a comfortable chair or while lying in bed.

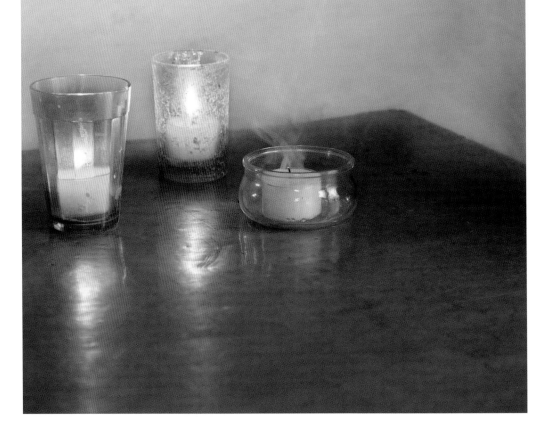

- Lie down flat on the floor and set a timer for five minutes.

- Place one hand on your tummy and one on your chest.

- Take a deep breath in through your nose. (If your nose is blocked, breathe through your mouth.) Try to breathe so that the hand on your tummy is the only one that initially moves. A good tip is to try to keep your shoulders relaxed as you are breathing. This helps encourage the breath to come from your diaphragm rather than your chest, which helps promote relaxation. You may find this a little tricky if you have never done this before. Keep practicing though, as this exercise becomes easier over time.

- When you feel as if you cannot easily take any more breath in with your tummy moving outwards, take in an extra bit— this final bit will come from your upper chest and, as you are taking it, you will feel the hand on your chest starting to move.

- Now breathe out fully, feeling your belly flatten as you do so. As you breathe out, both of your hands will be moving. This exhale should feel as if it takes a little bit longer than the inhale. Don't worry about timing this.

- Do this ten times.

- With each in-breath, pay attention to where the breath is coming in. For example, do you feel it through your nostrils, on your lips, or in your lungs? It doesn't matter which; the important thing is just to focus on the feeling of breath coming into your body.

- Do the same on the out-breath. Do you feel air rushing out of your nostrils on to your upper lip, or somewhere else? Focus on the sensation.

- As you go through the exercise you'll find that distracting thoughts will start to pop into your head. This is OK and fully to be expected. This happens to everyone, including experienced meditators.

- The idea is not to banish or block these thoughts. If you try to do this, you may well increase the tension in your body, which in turn can activate the body's stress response. Instead, simply acknowledge these thoughts and feelings. Watch them come and go in a spirit of detached curiosity. As soon as you notice that you've become distracted, slowly and smilingly return your attention to the breath.

- After ten breaths, return to a normal rhythm of breathing in and breathing out, continuing to notice where the breath is coming in and going out.

- Continue this process for a total of five minutes.

BREATH COUNTING

Practice being mindful by counting each of your out-breaths.

This is a simple technique inspired by methods used by practitioners of Zen Buddhism. It's particularly good if you struggle with concentrating for long periods or if you find it hard to pay attention. It is great for enhancing focus. The gentle practice of paying attention to your breath also helps you to become more mindful throughout the day. You might find it useful to make sure the airways in your nose are clear before you start.

- Sit upright in your chair and set a timer for five minutes. Make sure your back is comfortably straight.

- Take a few deep breaths in and out through your nose (or through your mouth if your nose is blocked).

- Now, allow the breath to return to its normal rate and rhythm.

- On the first exhale, count "1" inside your head. On the second exhale, count "2" inside your head. Keep counting on every exhale until you get to "5." Try to stay focused on your breathing the entire time.

- Once you get to "5," start counting again from "1" on the next exhale. Once again, continue counting on each exhale until you get to "5." Keep repeating this cycle, over and over again.

- If you feel your mind has wandered and you've stopped counting, don't worry. It's completely natural and a part of the process. Gently and lovingly acknowledge what has happened, go back to "1," and start counting again.

- Sometimes your mind might wander for quite some time and you'll find yourself counting beyond "5." I once went all the way to "30" before I realized what had happened. This is also fine. Once you're aware that your mind has wandered, gently return your attention to the breath and start from "1" again.

- Do this for five minutes.

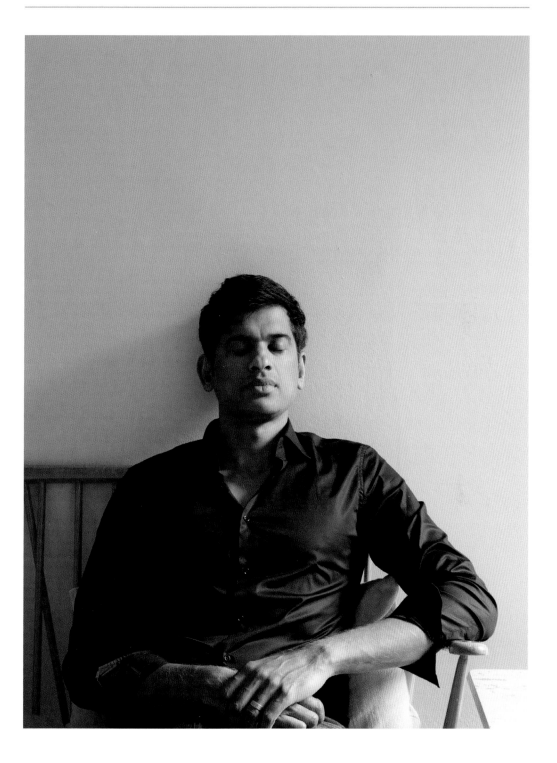

CASE STUDY

For years, forty-two-year-old Surinder had been suffering with pain in her legs and upper arms. The strong painkillers she'd been prescribed gave her constipation and made her drowsy, and she was getting more and more frustrated. Chronic pain is a notoriously tricky problem to manage and can be challenging to get on top of. But I wanted to start by trying to enable her to cope with it better. A big part of the problem was that Surinder didn't know when the pain was going to strike. This unpredictability meant she felt she could never relax. It affected her mood, the way she viewed life, and her close relationships.

Over the previous six months she found she'd become increasingly reclusive. She used to be incredibly social but, because she was either in pain or anxious about the pain kicking in, she found herself irritable and withdrawn when in the company of her friends. The same dynamics were happening at home, which caused inevitable strain with her children and husband.

There's good evidence to suggest that deep breathing can help change our perception of pain. I suggested that, as soon as she got back into the house after taking her kids to school, she spent five minutes doing the lying-down breathing practice outlined on page 95. After around three weeks she reported that her pain levels had come down by about half, which was incredible.

But that was only the start of it. Because she felt so much better, she felt happier. She could also take fewer painkillers, which made her less drowsy and decreased the discomfort from constipation. She started walking to a café every day and made some new friends among the other moms who went there regularly, which cheered her up even further. It was a classic Ripple Effect (page 25). One small health snack triggered a series of positive, unexpected benefits.

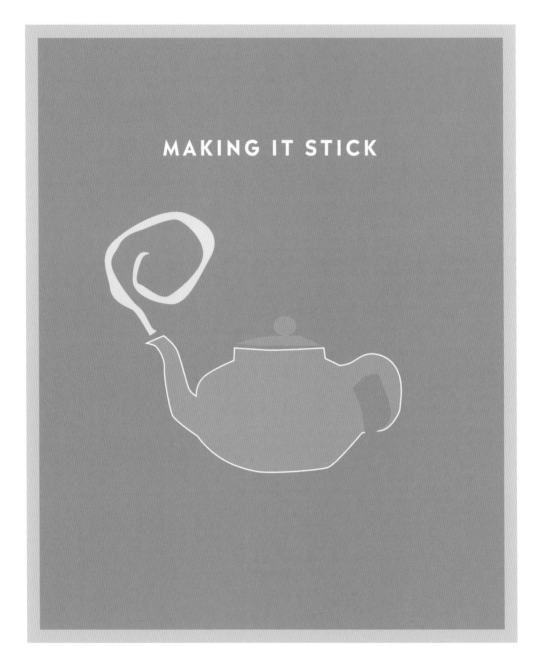

MAKING IT STICK

It's really important to pay attention to how you feel after your Breathe health snack. A critical part of making any new habit stick is really luxuriating in that feeling of reward once you've finished. So take a few quiet moments to internalize that feeling of calm, stillness, and relaxation that will hopefully be swimming about inside you like warm soup. Once you start to associate this new activity with the reward of feeling good, you'll begin to create a powerful association in the brain. Do it enough, and you'll begin craving the sensation, and craving the snack.

As with all the health snacks, I'd encourage you to stick this habit on to an existing daily routine. Some of my patients do a Breathe health snack in their bed as soon as they wake up. One likes to drink extremely strong-brewed tea every morning. She'd boil the kettle, put her tea to brew in a teapot, and, while it was brewing, she would do her five minutes of breathing. Her "reward" for doing it was her mug of tea.

You could always combine this health snack with another one from a different section of the book. I will often start my own day with five minutes of deep breathing, followed by a five-minute bodyweight workout (see page 119). I "stick" these two habits on to the start of my day and it means that within ten minutes of waking up, I have done two out of my three health snacks. It leaves me feeling energized and motivated and results in me being more productive for the rest of the day.

NOURISH

It might seem strange that I'm talking about nourishment in a section that's supposed to be about mental wellness, but over the last few years researchers have begun to find a surprisingly powerful connection between what we put in our mouths and how we feel in our heads. We've known for a very long time that nutrition is incredibly important for our bodies and our weight. We now know that it's just as important for looking after our minds.

Many foods contain nutrients that directly help improve the function of our brains. But, on top of this, there's also a direct pathway between our digestive system and our brains along which critical information about our wellbeing is constantly flowing. This pathway is sometimes called the "gut-brain axis." To understand how it works, you need to know that when we eat anything, we're not only feeding ourselves but also trillions of bacteria that live mostly in our large intestines. These "gut bugs" are crucial to our health because they process much of what we eat for us and produce by-products that can help us feel better. When these gut bugs are happy, this will be communicated up the gut–brain axis and we'll feel good. Our mood will improve. But when we make less helpful food choices, the reverse can happen.

Food is so much more than just energy or calories. It's actually information. If you provide good information to your gut bugs, they will then communicate that to your brain and send calming signals. But if you give them food that they don't like, they will send stress signals. Many modern highly processed foods can have a terrible effect on our gut bugs, wiping them out by the millions. In addition, anything that contains artificial additives, emulsifiers, pesticides, or chemical sweeteners has the potential to negatively affect them. Even many popular medications, including antibiotics and bestselling heartburn medications, can play havoc with our gut bugs that can take months to recover from.

This health snack really is an actual snack. I'm going to give you a variety of options to nourish your mind so that, on every Feel Better Day, you'll be providing your gut bugs with the right nutrients and your brain with the right information.

Our brains thrive on certain nutrients. The problem is, many of us struggle to find the time to create healthy home-cooked meals. If this sounds like you, a five-minute smoothie can make a real difference.

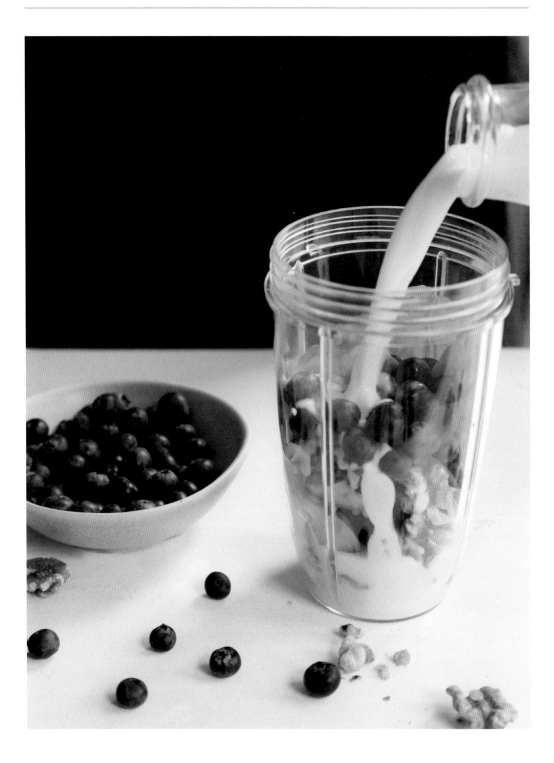

MIND THE BLUEBERRIES

Spend five minutes making yourself a delicious brain-nourishing smoothie.

Throw my favorite brain-nourishing nutrients into a blender and blitz until smooth.

½ cup blueberries (frozen is fine)

half an avocado

2 handfuls of leafy greens (e.g., spinach or kale)

1 tablespoon of coconut oil

handful of walnuts

cacao powder (optional, for taste)

unsweetened almond milk or water

- **Blueberries** are rich in fiber, loaded with healthy phytonutrients and antioxidants, and research has shown that they are good for brain function and memory.

- **Avocados** are a great source of the healthy fats our brain needs to work at its best.

- **Dark green leafy vegetables** are full of vitamins, minerals, and fiber that are essential for a well-functioning nervous system.

- **Coconut oil** tastes fantastic and contains a kind of fat that can be directly used as fuel by the brain.

- **Walnuts** are rich in a type of fat called omega 3, which is known to be important for optimal brain function. In addition, they are rich in helpful polyphenols, antioxidants, and vitamin E, and observational studies have shown that walnut eaters have better brain function.

FB
LM

You can listen to me talk about the amazing power of blueberries as well as other foods that help to feed the brain in my *Feel Better, Live More* podcast conversation with Dr. Lisa Mosconi at drchatterjee.com/lisamosconi

HAPPY BRAIN SMOOTHIE

Spend five minutes nourishing your "gut-brain axis" with this delicious smoothie.

Throw these gut-enhancing ingredients into a blender and blitz until smooth.

¾ cup milk (cow's, goat's, or unsweetened plant milk, e.g., almond)

3 tablespoons kefir

1 heaping tablespoon almond butter (or peanut butter)

1 small avocado

6–8 raspberries

½ tablespoon 100% cacao powder

¼ teaspoon ground cinnamon

¼ teaspoon ground turmeric or ½-inch fresh turmeric root

1 teaspoon psyllium husks or ½ teaspoon ground psyllium husk (optional)

a pinch of ground ginger or ¼-inch fresh ginger root (optional)

- **Kefir** is lovely and creamy and provides you with a source of live bacteria or "probiotics" that can help improve your gut health.

- **Almond butter** contains biotin, which is essential for the health of your gut barrier; zinc, which supports brain health; and magnesium, which helps give you more energy.

- **Raspberries** are a rich source of polyphenols, which feed your gut bugs and help them produce short-chain fatty acids that can help support brain health.

- **Cacao powder** is a source of flavanols, which are known to support the heart and to potentially help our brains as well.

- **Cinnamon** helps improve brain health by helping you balance blood sugar levels and contains particular polyphenols that help the brain stay young.

- **Turmeric** is a source of curcumin, a natural substance, that feeds gut bacteria and has beneficial effects on the brain.

- **Psyllium** (optional) is a soluble fiber that results in low gas production, so it is great for those with a tendency to bloat.

- **Ginger** (optional) is a source of gingerols, which are anti-inflammatory and can help calm upset stomachs.

This smoothie has been created by the brilliant neuroscientist, nutritionist, and expert in the gut-brain axis, Miguel Toribio-Mateas (@miguelmateas). Listen to my conversation with him on my *Feel Better, Live More* podcast at drchatterjee.com/miguel

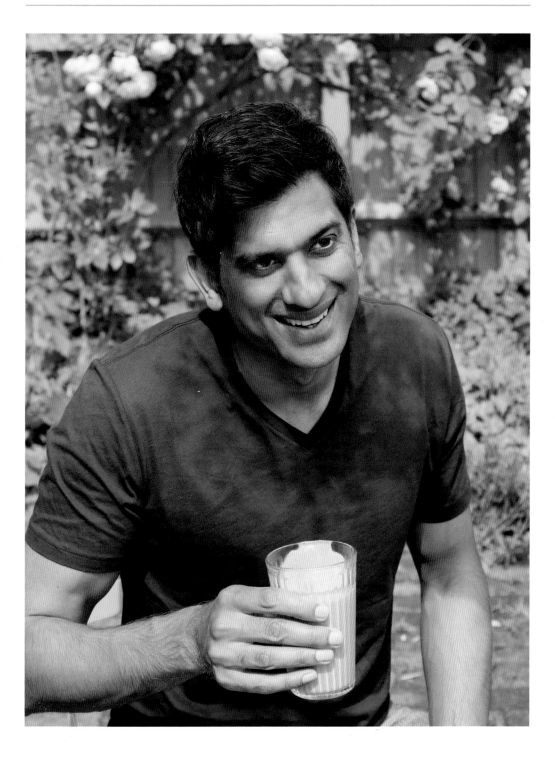

THE GUT BUGS HEALTH SNACK

Feed your gut bugs the foods they love.

Your gut bugs love the fiber that's found in bright, colorful vegetables. No matter what food tribe you might subscribe to, whether you're vegan, low-carb, paleo, or a passionate meat-eater, pretty much all mainstream nutritionists agree that eating more veg is a good thing. Why not spend five minutes each day focusing on giving your gut bugs a tasty but healthy snack that they will love?

- Chop up some of your favorite vegetables to either eat now or take with you for a snack later on when you are out and about.

- Carrots, cucumber, peppers, celery, radishes, etc. work especially well.

- If eating immediately, you can team them with your favorite type of nut butter or hummus for a delicious and healthy snack that will also help you nourish your mind.

FB LM You can listen to a detailed conversation between myself and Professor Tim Spector on gut health at drchatterjee.com/timspector

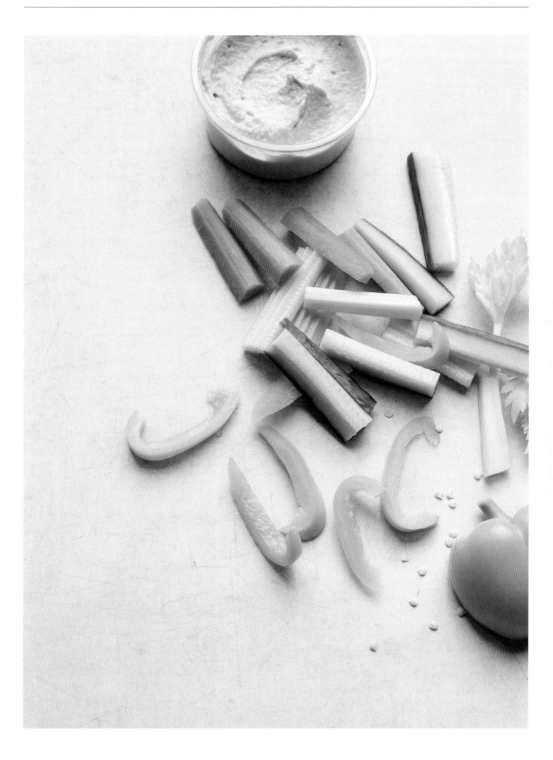

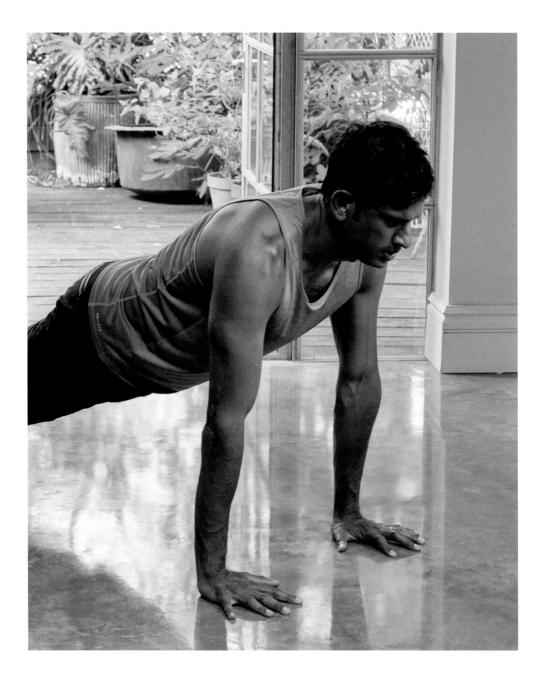

2
BODY

FIVE MINUTES OF MOVEMENT ON EACH OF
YOUR "FEEL BETTER DAYS" WILL QUICKLY
TRANSFORM YOUR LIFE

BODY SNACKS MENU

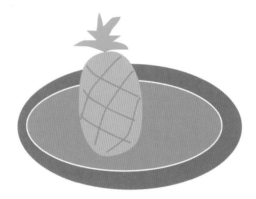

CHOOSE **ONE** HEALTH SNACK
TO **GET YOUR BODY MOVING**

STRENGTH

THE CLASSIC 5

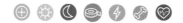

SWEAT

THE POWER 5 | SIMPLE SWEAT | THE EASY KNEESY | THE HIIT SQUAD

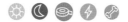

PLAY

JUST PLAY! | DANCING | JUMPING ROPE

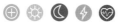

BALANCE

DESK JOCKEY WORKOUT | THE CLOCK WORKOUT

RESTORE

THE MORNING WAKE-UP FLOW | THE DAY'S END RELEASE FLOW

BODY

It doesn't surprise me that so many of us have an unhealthy relationship with our bodies these days. We're surrounded by images of what we're told is absolute physical perfection and are continually sold the idea that these kinds of bodies are both ordinary and attainable. If we think we fall short of these impossible ideals, we can so easily feel ashamed and start to beat ourselves up.

These images fill our television programs, our advertising, and our social media feeds. For a long time, I've noticed that they make a worrying number of people give up taking care of their physical health before they've even begun. I see so many patients who are carrying excess weight who believe that, because "Insta-perfection" is impossible to achieve, there's no point in doing anything at all. This is damaging, and it's completely wrong. It's crucial to understand that health isn't some faraway goal. If you're breathing, you already have health. But it's always good to have more of it, no matter where you're starting from.

So don't fall into the same trap as these people. Don't tell yourself that there's no point in doing any exercise if it isn't going to make you "beach body ready," or that working out only counts if it takes the form of an hour on the treadmill or a dizzying spin class or a five-mile run. It's simply not true.

It's absolutely critical for your overall wellbeing that you move your body regularly. Five minutes of focused exercise on each one of your Feel Better Days will quickly begin to add up and ultimately make a big difference to the way you feel. You'll be regularly making your heart pump faster and forcing your muscles to adapt to the extra strain that's being put on them. You'll also be moving blood around your body, which increases oxygen delivery to your cells and gives your joints what they really want—movement. Five minutes of movement on each of your Feel Better Days will quickly transform your life.

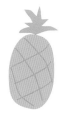

GLOSSARY

GLUTES

the muscles in your bottom

HAMSTRINGS

the muscles on the back of your thighs

QUADS

the muscles at the front of your thighs

CORE

the chain of deep abdominal muscles that helps to support your spine
(not "six-pack" muscles, which are superficial)

STRENGTH

When we think about strength training, our minds tend to picture images of over-tanned gods and goddesses in Lycra, their biceps bulging as they grunt and sweat beneath huge barbells. Many people find that the very idea of themselves weightlifting is silly or comical. This is a huge shame. The simple fact is, strength training definitely isn't just for posers and young, body-conscious people. Strength training is arguably the most undervalued component of fitness.

What many of us don't realize is that our muscles are more than just lumps of meat. They're not just there to move our bodies around. Our muscles are organs that contribute to the essential running of our system, just like our kidneys, heart, or liver do. They help manufacture the energy we need to live. As well as this, they act a bit like sponges to soak up the sugar our bodies naturally produce when we eat certain foods such as bread, pasta, and potatoes. Strength training is a critical weapon in our battle against the development of type 2 diabetes, a disease that's thought to affect as many as thirty-two million people in the US alone. It also helps us burn more calories throughout the day, to maintain a healthy weight, to build stronger bones, and to improve our mood.

The older you are, the more you stand to benefit from strength training. After the age of about thirty we naturally start losing muscle, which means we need to work on our strength just to maintain what we had. And the older we get, the more muscle we lose. By the time we hit our fifties, our muscle power is dropping at a rate of around 3 percent every year. Not

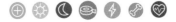

only are these valuable organs shrinking and weakening, they're changing in form, becoming more marbled with fat. This will have a negative consequence on levels of important hormones such as growth hormone and testosterone, which are needed for us to grow new muscle and make strong bones. All this means we have less ability to do the normal activities of day-to-day life, whether it's carrying our groceries into the house or playing in the park with our kids or grandkids.

Regular strength training reverses aging in many of our most important muscles and increases the amount of mitochondria our bodies have. Mitochondria are the body's energy factories, so having more of them can help fight fatigue. The more of it you do, the more lean muscle mass you'll build, and lean muscle mass is one of the most powerful predictors of a long and healthy life. This means that, as you get older, you'll be more active, more mobile, and will get tired less easily.

Because this kind of training is so incredibly beneficial, I've designed the Strength health snacks in *Feel Better in 5* so that they're as straight-forward as possible. They don't require a visit to the gym, any exotic or expensive equipment, and can be modified to suit any ability level. You don't even need to get changed to do them. You should be able to do them in your kitchen or bedroom, and none of them will take any more than five minutes to complete.

 You can listen to a conversation on my *Feel Better, Live More* podcast about the importance of strength at drchatterjee.com/strength

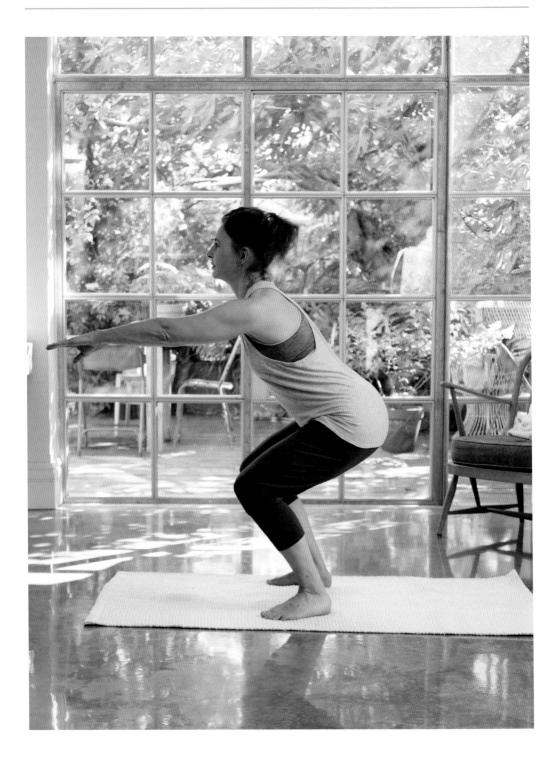

THE CLASSIC 5

Become stronger with this no-equipment whole-body workout.

This is a sequence of classic bodyweight exercises that'll give all the major muscles in your body a workout. They're also accessible to virtually anyone. I have patients in their twenties and all the way up to their eighties regularly practicing this workout. They are simply the best five exercises that can be done with no equipment at all—meaning there is very little reason not to do them.

They will certainly help you tone your body, but they are not just vanity exercises—they work on the muscles and movement patterns that you need to function well in everyday life. They will help you feel better about yourself, increase your confidence, increase your energy, help reduce pain and niggles, enable you to walk, cycle, or run farther, and allow you to play for longer with any children (or grandchildren!) you may have.

LUNGES

REVERSE FLY

SQUATS

PUSH-UPS

GLUTE BRIDGES

Do each of these exercises for thirty seconds, one after the other. Repeat the entire sequence two times—this will take you only five minutes!

There's no need to have a break after each exercise as they all work different parts of the body. However, if you do need a short break of ten seconds or so between each exercise, that's fine. If you are unable to go the full thirty seconds on one particular exercise, that is also fine. Just stop and move on to the next exercise when the thirty seconds is up.

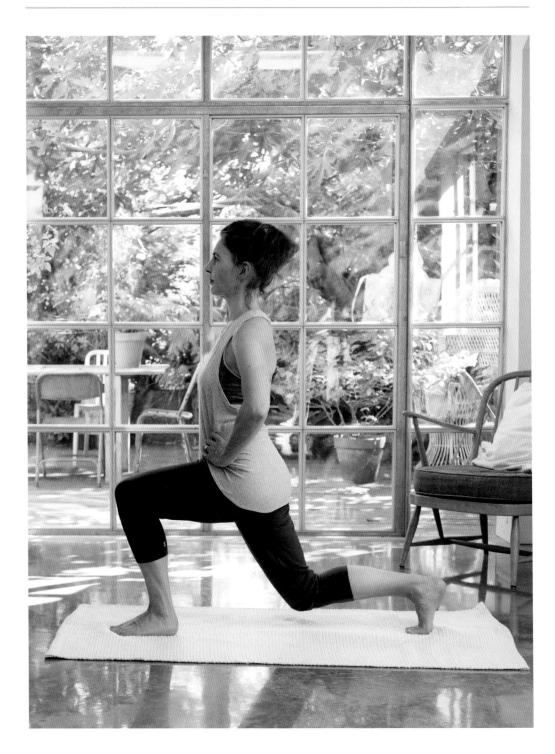

LUNGE

Lunges are a fabulous way of strengthening your glutes, quads, and hamstrings. They also build up your balance and work on your hip flexibility. There are many different ways to do a lunge. If you have never done lunges before, I would recommend that you start with the reverse lunge.

Reverse lunge

- Stand upright with your feet shoulder width apart, placing your hands on your hips.

- Step back with your right foot and bend both knees. Keep your right heel off the ground and aim to create 90-degree angles between your thighs and shins.

- Try to keep your chest as upright as you can. You'll feel as if your glutes and quad muscles are being worked.

- Push through the heel of your left foot to return to standing.

- Do 15 seconds on each leg. This will make up your full 30 seconds for your lunges. (If you prefer, you can do your first 30 seconds on one leg and when you are going through the five exercises for the second time, you can do 30 seconds on your other leg.)

- Now move on to the next exercise.

Once you are comfortable doing the reverse lunge, you can make the exercise more challenging by doing a **forward lunge**—instead of lunging by stepping back behind you, you would step forward and lunge out in front of you. Remember to keep your upper body straight and your front knee directly above your ankle. (The photo opposite works for both lunges as the end position looks the same.)

The reverse lunge and forward lunge are slightly different movements. Feel free to do them both and mix it up from workout to workout, if you wish.

As you get stronger, an excellent progression is to move continuously from a forward lunge to a reverse lunge and back again without putting your foot down halfway. Remember to do both legs.

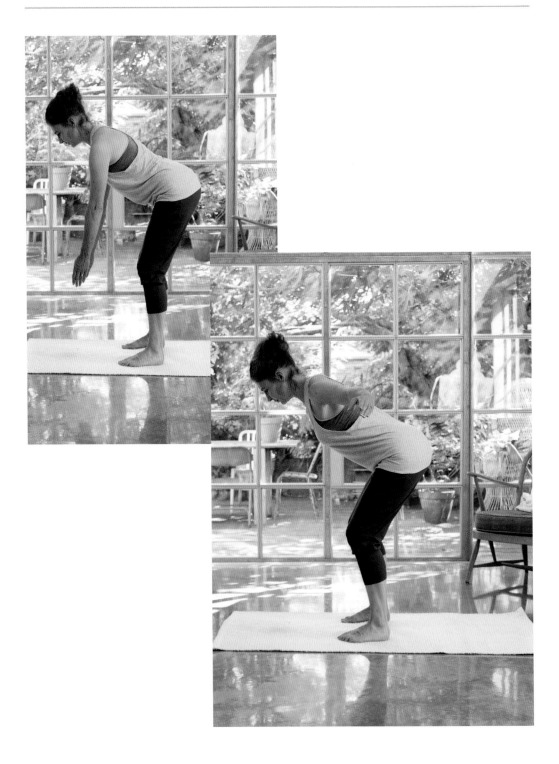

REVERSE FLY

This exercise is great for those of us who sit at desks all day hunched over a computer screen. It targets the shoulders and upper-back muscles and is fantastic for posture.

- Lean forward at the waist. Use a hinging motion so that your back remains straight. Your knees should have a slight bend in them and your arms should hang towards the floor.

- Bring both arms upwards and outwards to the side until you feel your shoulder blades touching each other. Stay in this position for two to three seconds.

- Now return slowly to the starting position, remaining in control of your movements.

- Do not use momentum or a swinging action to lift your arms.

- After 30 seconds, move on to the next exercise.

To make it harder, simply pick up some cans of beans, bottles of water, or light dumbbells and hold in each hand.

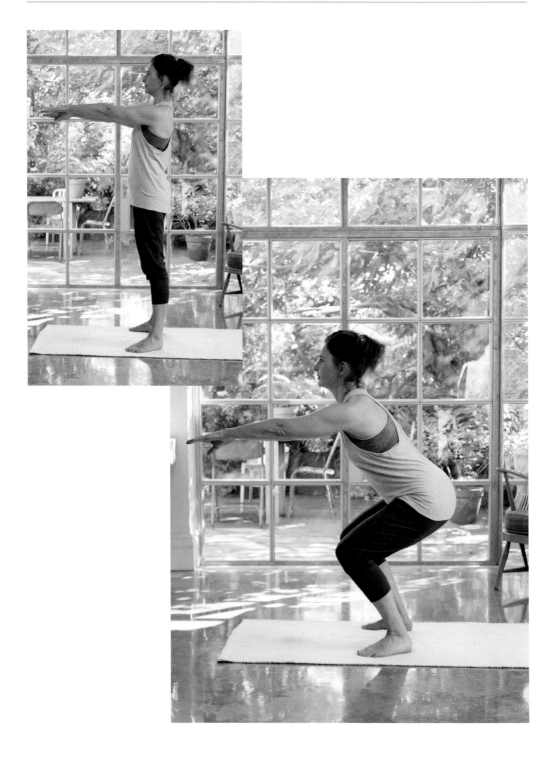

SQUATS

A squat is a whole-body movement that you may feel most in your glutes and quads but it also helps to build balance and coordination. The ultimate goal is to be able to squat all the way down so your bottom is almost touching the ground. However, this requires a level of ankle and hip flexibility that few of us have these days. With regular practice, however, your strength and mobility will improve.

- Start in a standing position with your feet slightly turned out and a little wider than hip width apart.

- Put your arms out in front of you to help with balance. If you need extra support, you can hold on to a chair or table.

- Start to lower yourself towards the floor, bottom first, as if you're sitting down.

- Gently inhale as you move your hips back and bend your knees.

- Try to keep your back straight and your chest as open as you can. It can be helpful to look straight ahead of you rather than at the floor below.

- Make sure that your knees are following the line of your feet as you go down.

- Go as far down as you can comfortably manage. Over time, you will be able to squat deeper.

- Drive your heels into the ground and, as you exhale, squeeze your glutes to push yourself back up to the starting position.

- After 30 seconds, move on to the next exercise.

To make the exercise harder, try squatting with your hands behind your head. You can also progress to doing them while holding some cans of beans, bottles of water, or light dumbbells in each hand.

When you are feeling really strong (as you will do with regular practice!), you can always have a go at a one-legged squat.

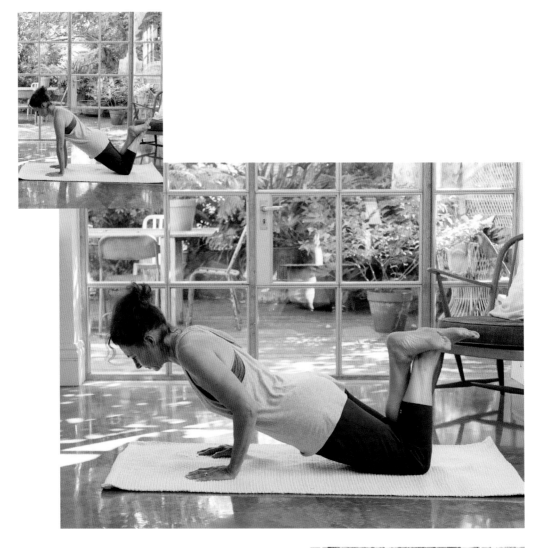

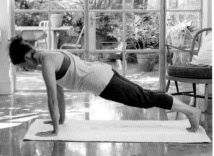

The "classic" push-up is done with knees
off the ground and feet on the floor.

PUSH-UPS

When done properly, push-ups work on your chest, arms, tummy muscles, and even your glutes. Doing them on the floor is actually pretty tough. Many of my patients start with their knees on the floor. If that is too challenging, you can start against a wall, a table, or kitchen countertop (see page 129). Start off at a level where you can comfortably perform the movement for 30 seconds.

- Start with your palms on the floor, shoulder width apart, and your knees touching the ground. If needed, pop a cushion under your knees and feel free to cross your feet if more comfortable (see photo opposite).

- As you breathe in, lower your body by bending your elbows, ensuring that your body remains in a straight line from head to knees. Keep your elbows tucked in to reduce the strain on your shoulders.

- Go as far down as you can comfortably manage. Feel as if your shoulder blades are pressing together when you're as low as you can go.

- As you push back up, breathe out and return to the starting position.

- After 30 seconds, move on to the next exercise.

THREE TIPS TO HELP TECHNIQUE

1 As you go down, feel as if you are screwing your hands into the ground, the left hand counter-clockwise and right hand clockwise. This helps to keep your shoulders in the correct position.

2 Feel your stomach muscles tense and squeeze your glutes as you go down. This helps to keep your body straight and in the correct position.

3 As you are moving down, try to keep your forearms at approximately 90 degrees to the floor. You may have to move your hands back a little to achieve this.

Once you are able to do "classic" push-ups for 30 seconds, you can make them harder by placing your feet on an elevated surface or by adding in a clap in between each push-up.

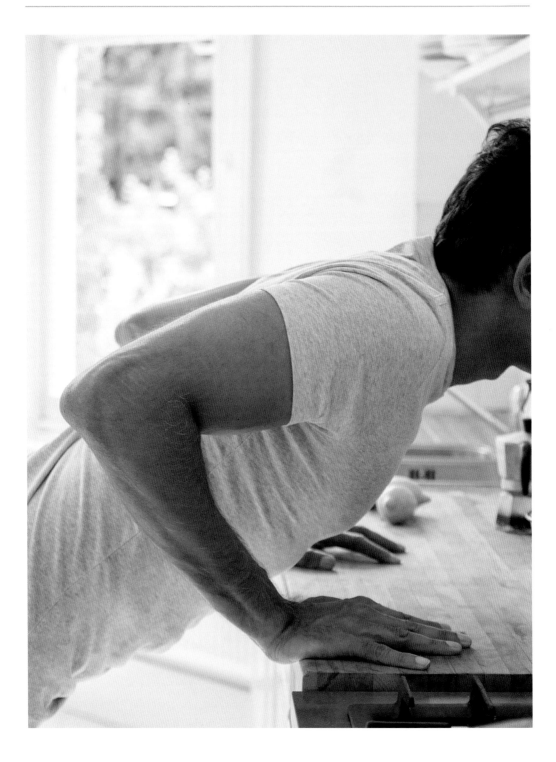

HOW TO CHANGE THE DIFFICULTY OF A PUSH-UP

There are seemingly endless ways to do push-ups, making them suitable for all ability levels. Here are a few common variations:

AGAINST A WALL

This is the easiest way to start. Stand approximately arm's length away from the wall and set your hands down just wider than shoulder width apart. As you bend your elbows, move your body towards the wall until your nose almost touches it. At the same time, squeeze your glutes and tense your stomach muscles, as this will help keep your body in a straight line. Straighten your arms to return your body to the starting position.

AGAINST AN ELEVATED SURFACE

This is slightly harder than a wall push-up and is a great way to progress when you feel ready. Place your hands on an elevated surface, like a kitchen countertop, as in the photo opposite. Bend your elbows to lower yourself down, while keeping your body straight. To make the movement harder, bring the height of the elevated surface down, e.g., from a kitchen countertop down to a dining table.

KNEES ON THE GROUND

Slightly harder still is to do a push-up with both knees on the ground. (See instructions and pictures on pages 126–7.) Once you can comfortably perform knees-on-the-ground push-ups with good form, you may be ready to move up to the regular "classic" push-up, where you have your knees off the ground and feet on the floor.

In a "classic" push-up you lift 64 percent of your bodyweight. With a knees-on-the-ground push-up, you lift approximately 49 percent of your bodyweight. If you put your hands on a 24-inch-high bench, you lift 41 percent. If you put your hands on a 36-inch-high surface (a bit higher than most kitchen surfaces), you lift 20 percent of your bodyweight. If you do a classic push-up with your feet elevated on a 24-inch-high bench, it increases to 75 percent.

There is always a variation that will work for your current strength levels!

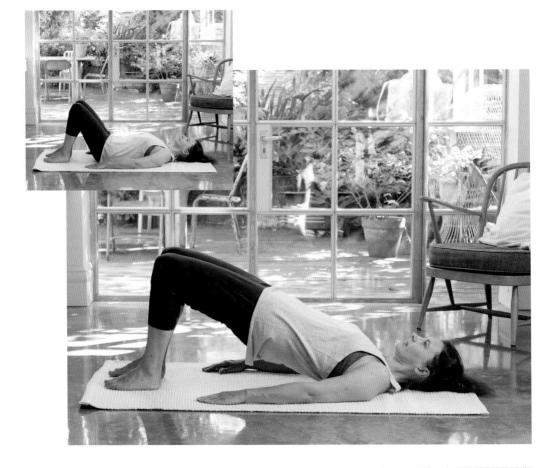

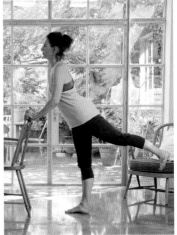

GLUTE BRIDGE

Glute bridges work on your glutes, hamstrings, hips, lower-back muscles, and core. They are what we call a "functional" exercise, which means they are particularly good at helping you in many of your day-to-day movements, such as carrying the shopping, going up stairs, and bending down to lift objects from the floor.

- Lie face up on the floor with your knees bent and your hands palms down by your side.

- Keeping your back straight, feel as if your stomach muscles are tightening, squeeze your bottom muscles and lift your hips up off the floor.

- Return to the starting position, with control. It can be helpful to count to three as you lower yourself back down.

- After 30 seconds, if this is your first time through the exercises, go back to the beginning of The Classic 5.

To make this harder, you can try to do the movement with only one leg on the floor. From the starting position, lift one foot off the ground until your thigh is at 90 degrees to the floor. Now try to lift your hips up off the floor using only one leg.

ALTERNATIVE STANDING GLUTE EXTENSION

Many of my patients have asked me to provide them with a glute bridge alternative for when the floor they are on is a bit hard or mucky—for example, a kitchen or office. I want to make sure you have no excuses to avoid doing this health snack!

- Hold on to the back of a chair or elevated surface, like a kitchen worktop. This is your starting position.

- Lift your left leg off the ground and move it back behind you without arching your back. You will start to feel your left glute muscle contract. From this position, turn your left foot out slightly

- to deepen the contraction. Hold this position for a maximum of 5 seconds.

- Return your left leg to the starting position.

- Repeat the movement on the right leg.

- Alternate 5 seconds on each leg until your 30 seconds is up.

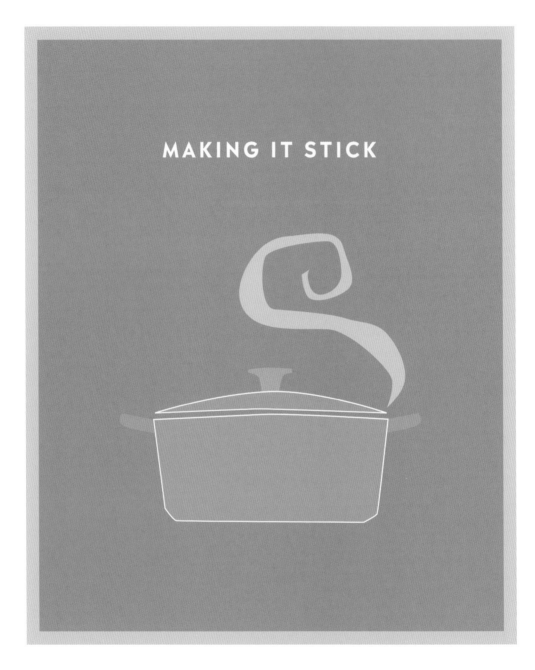

MAKING IT STICK

Motivation comes and goes in waves, which is why you cannot rely on it to make long-term change. When you start this program, no doubt your motivation will be high. Use this high level of motivation to learn one of the Body workouts, like The Classic 5. Once you have done it for a few days, you will be able to complete the whole workout without much thought, and without referring to this book. At this stage, the health snack will feel relatively easy. This will come in very handy on those days when your motivation is low. Research tells us that when our motivation is high, we are able to do behaviors that feel hard, but when motivation is low, we will only do our new behavior if it feels easy.

As with all new habits, it really helps to do your Strength health snack at the same time and in the same place every day. Many of my patients love to do theirs in the kitchen. Most of us are in our kitchens at least once during the day. Often in the morning to make a cup of coffee or in the evening before dinner. These are the perfect times to do a Strength workout.

Why not make it a plan that you'll do your Strength workout every day before dinner? Before you know it, you will be doing these new behaviors without thinking. They will have become automatic. They will have become new habits.

SWEAT

I'm a huge fan of taking my exercise in short, sharp bursts. Not only is it much more convenient and affordable than sweating it out in a long session at the gym, it's also surprisingly effective. Over the last few years there's been a lot of interest in what's known as High Intensity Interval Training, or HIIT. This usually involves pushing yourself physically for less than a minute, having a short break to recover, then repeating again and again.

Researchers who've studied the effects of HIIT have found that it's good for your muscles, your brain and your bones. It also helps your mitochondria, which are the tiny power-packs that give the cells in your body their energy. It even helps your body's sensitivity to the hormone insulin, which lowers your chances of suffering with type 2 diabetes.

If all that wasn't enough, HIIT also attacks an especially dangerous kind of fat known as "visceral fat." This is a type of fat that covers our internal organs and is linked with increased rates of type 2 diabetes, strokes, and heart attacks. One part of the reason visceral fat is such a problem is that, because it lives on the inside of our bodies, it's largely invisible. In fact, it's quite common for people to look thin but actually be carrying dangerous levels of visceral fat in their bodies. These men and women are sometimes referred to as being TOFI—thin on the outside, fat on the inside. The great thing about HIIT is that it's much better at targeting visceral fat than more conventional workouts.

I've created a few five-minute HIIT workouts for you to choose from. If you're based at home during the week you can do them at any time of the day, but I'd recommend exercising just before lunch as this will change the way your body processes your meal for the better. But if you're not at home and are worrying about getting sweaty during your lunch hour, then getting your HIIT health snack in before your evening meal or even before

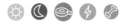

breakfast will reward you with the same benefits. Once you get into the habit of doing these five-minute workouts on each of your Feel Better Days, the way you feel about yourself will change, your energy levels will improve, and you'll start to notice changes in your body shape.

HERE IS YOUR HIIT WORKOUT PRESCRIPTION:

BEGINNER:

20 seconds on, 40 seconds off **x 5**

INTERMEDIATE:

30 seconds on, 30 seconds off **x 5**

ADVANCED:

40 seconds on, 20 seconds off **x 5**

Start at the level that suits your current fitness levels and, as you get stronger, you'll soon find you're able to increase the amount of time you're exercising and reduce your periods of rest.

THE POWER 5

Perform five quick exercises in just five minutes to work your entire body.

This workout is a simple way to get all the benefits of HIIT training while working on different areas of the body at the same time.

JOGGING ON THE SPOT

JUMPING JACKS

MOUNTAIN CLIMBERS

PUSH-UPS

SUMO SQUATS

These five movements should be completed one after the other in the prescribed time intervals on the previous page.

If you find you can't do one or more of these exercises because it feels too hard, is causing pain, or because you have an injury, you can easily substitute another exercise, even if it means repeating one of them. You can even do the Simple Sweat workout (page 143), where you choose one of the above five exercises that you enjoy and can do easily and simply repeat it over and over again for the prescribed time intervals.

Don't look for reasons not to do the workout. I have designed this program to be as simple and accessible as possible—there is always a way!

JOGGING ON THE SPOT

Jog from foot to foot, staying on the same spot on the floor.

Go as hard as you can for the duration of your exercise.

You should feel out of breath by the time you get to your rest period.

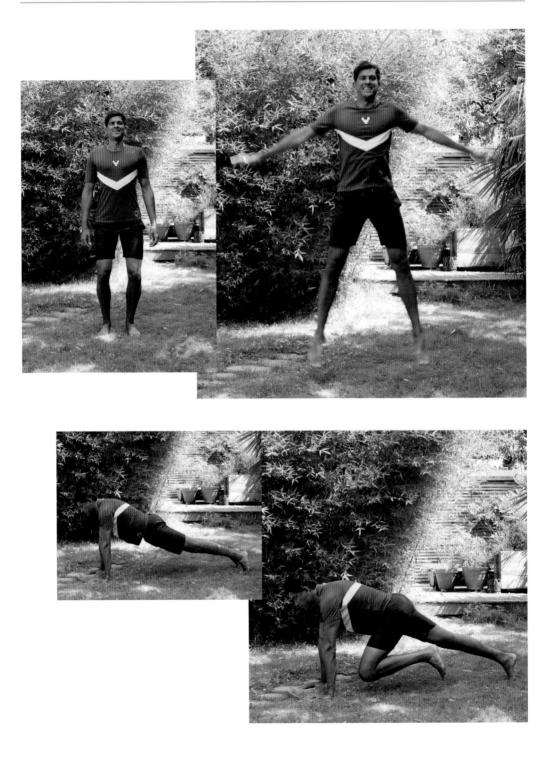

JUMPING JACKS

- Stand up straight in a relaxed stance with your feet close together and your arms close to your body.

- Jump up and out, so that your feet land wider than hip width apart and your arms rise out to the side.

- Jump back to the starting position by bringing your feet together and your arms down by your sides.

- Repeat this movement as many times as you can within the prescribed time interval.

MOUNTAIN CLIMBERS

- Place yourself in a traditional push-up position. Your hands should be directly under your shoulders and you should feel as if your pelvis is being tucked under your body so the arch in your lower back disappears.

- Try to make sure your body is perfectly aligned, with your head, shoulders, and bottom all in one straight line.

- Bring your left knee forward until it is underneath your chest.

- Return your left leg to the starting position and switch legs.

- Continue, quickly alternating between legs: this is a fast movement.

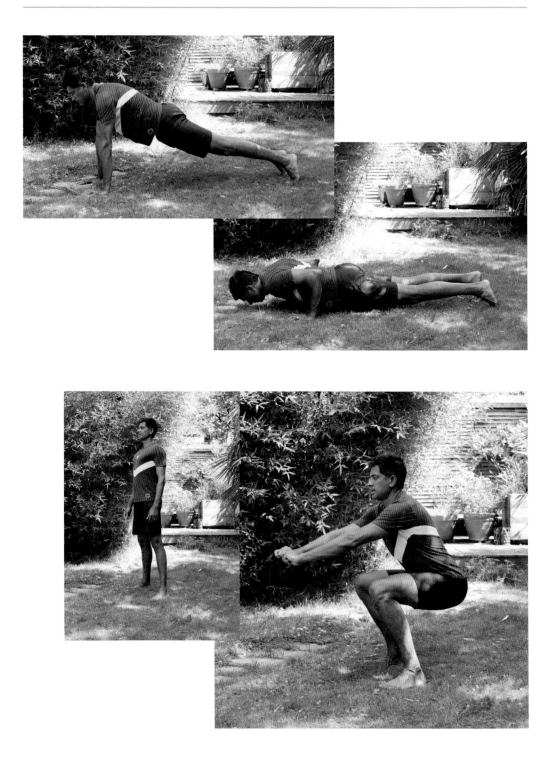

PUSH-UPS

- Start with your palms on the floor, shoulder width apart, and your feet touching the ground.

- Lower your body by bending your elbows, ensuring that your body remains in a straight line from head to toe.

- Keep your elbows tucked in. Flaring your elbows out to the side puts a lot of strain on your shoulders.

- As you go down, breathe in. Go as far down as you can comfortably manage. Feel as if your shoulder blades are pressing together when you're as low as you can go.

- As you push back up, breathe out and return to the starting position.

Remember, you can easily alter the difficulty of a push-up to suit your current ability level (see page 129).

SUMO SQUATS

- Stand with your feet a bit wider than hip width apart and turned out a little.

- Bend your knees and lower your body down as if sitting in a chair behind you. Feel your weight go into your heels. If you need extra support, hold on to the back of a chair or table.

- Keep going down as far as you can and stop if you manage to get your thighs parallel to the ground.

- Squeeze the muscles in your bottom as you come back up and return to your standing position.

- Throughout the exercise, make sure your chest is up and out and that your knees track your toes as you go down.

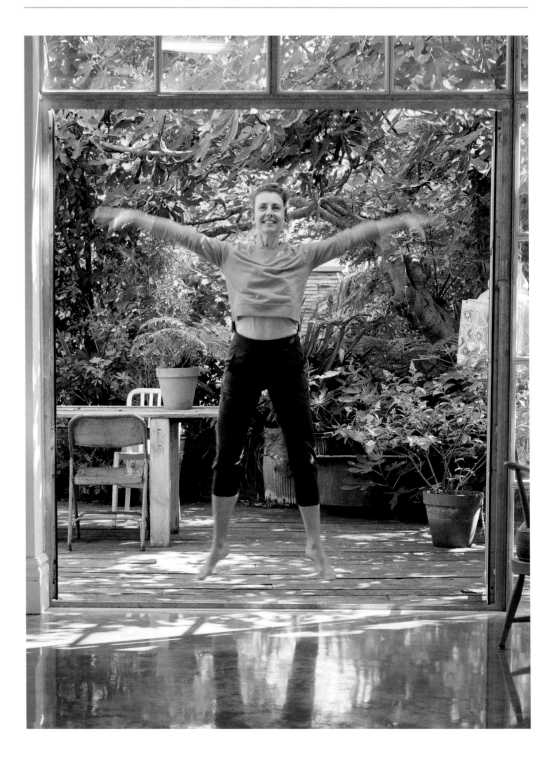

SIMPLE SWEAT

Choose one exercise you love and repeat for five quick intervals.

This is the easiest way I know of getting your five minutes of Sweat in on your Feel Better Days. It doesn't require much space, skill, time, or money. It certainly doesn't mean hiring a personal trainer or joining a gym. It's simply a case of choosing just one exercise that gets your heart pumping.

Take a look at the five choices in The Power 5 health snack on page 136 and select one. I'd particularly recommend jumping jacks, as they work your upper and lower body at the same time.

CHOOSE YOUR FAVORITE EXERCISE FROM THE POWER 5

Once you've made your choice, repeat the exercise for the prescribed amount of time. For example, if you are a beginner, push yourself as hard as you can for twenty seconds, stop for forty seconds and repeat five times. As you get fitter, you can increase the exercise time and reduce the rest time.

(One of my patients is in tip-top physical condition and his entire exercise regime consists *only* of doing this 5 minute workout; Monday to Friday; as soon as he gets home from work!)

CASE STUDY

Hui Yin was a thirty-eight-year-old HR manager who had been trying to get pregnant with her husband for about two years. She was very proactive about her health and had been since school. As a teenager, she'd been a prize-winning long-distance runner. These days, she'd get up at five in the morning to go to the gym on the way to work, where she'd exercise for an hour, and she'd also play squash in the evening. She took her job seriously and was proud of her ability to deal with pressure at work.

There was no obvious reason why she couldn't conceive. Her blood tests all came back normal and her lifestyle was fairly healthy. Her husband had a child from a previous relationship and all his fertility tests were fine. I began to wonder if she might be exercising too much. Too much exercise can put a significant amount of stress on the body, and I have seen, on many occasions, this having a negative impact on a woman's fertility.

I asked Hui Yin if she would consider stopping going to the gym. This came as a complete shock to her. She thought her daily hard exercise had been helping her. I could also tell that the gym was part of her identity. It was how she felt good about herself. But I was worried that it was too much for her, on top of long hours in a very stressful job.

I suggested that she swap out her intense gym sessions for just five minutes of daily yoga at home. I told her that I thought she was burning out and that her intense workouts were putting too much stress on her body. I explained that yoga would be more restorative for her and recommended that she do her five minutes in the evening, so she'd have more time in bed in the mornings.

Two weeks later she was back. Hui Yin had tried yoga, and she hated it. She was back at the gym, every single day. I realized, once again, that the best health interventions are usually the ones that fold around a patient's life, not the other way around. It was the endorphin rush that Hui Yin was addicted to and, for all its benefits, yoga was not going to provide that—at least, not yet.

But I knew something that would. When I suggested five minutes of HIIT, she was so relieved I wasn't insisting on more yoga that she promised to give it a go straight away. Thankfully, she loved it. She'd come home from work and push herself to her limit, burn off the stress of the day and feel that her muscles were getting toned, which was something that was very important to her. When I saw her six weeks later she looked every bit as fit as she did before but she looked more healthy. The bags under her eyes were gone, there was color in her cheeks, and she just had a zip and zing she previously lacked. Three months later Hui Yin was pregnant. I'd love to say that doing HIIT instead of over-exercising at the gym was behind this, but, of course, I can't be sure. I strongly suspect, however, it played a major role, and so does Hui Yin. I've also seen the same effects in several other women.

THE EASY KNEESY

I've created this low-impact workout for those of you who prefer to reduce the impact on your knees. Again, complete each of the following five movements, one after the other, in the prescribed time intervals specified on page 135.

> **HIGH KNEES WITH SHOULDER PRESS**
>
> **SQUAT WITH KNEE TO HAND**
>
> **STRAIGHT PUNCHES**
>
> **SITTING ARM PUNCH**
>
> **PUSH-UP ON KNEES**

HIGH KNEES WITH SHOULDER PRESS

- March on the spot, bringing your knees as high as you can.

- Each time one of your knees comes up, push both hands upwards towards the ceiling.

- As the knee returns to the ground, bring both arms down to your sides.

SQUAT WITH KNEE TO HAND

- Squat down as low as you can comfortably go with your arms out in front of you (see page 125 for detailed instructions).

- Come back up to standing. As you do so, lift your left knee up to touch your right hand.

- Do the same on the other side.

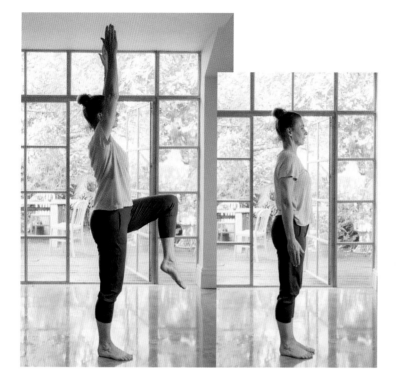

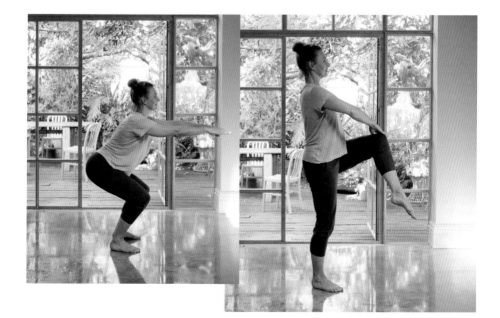

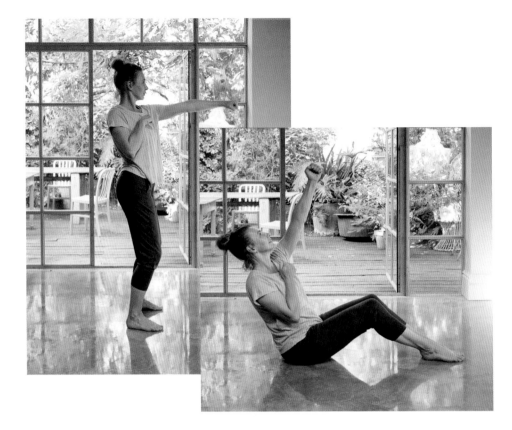

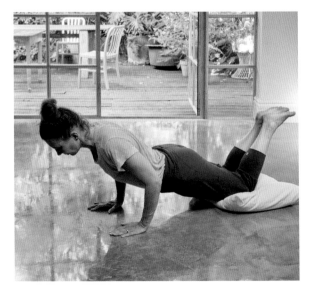

STRAIGHT PUNCHES

- Stand up straight with a very slight bend in your knees.

- Make a fist with both hands and bring up to your chest.

- Punch out each arm in front of you, alternating between left and right.

- Keep your arms level with your chest and look straight ahead.

SITTING ARM PUNCH

- Sit up on the ground with your knees bent in front of you and your feet flat on the floor.

- Lean back a little, until you feel your stomach muscles engage.

- Make sure you are feeling comfortable in this position. If it feels too hard, straighten back up a little.

- From this position, punch alternate arms into the air.

PUSH-UP ON KNEES

- Get down into a push-up position but drop both knees to the floor. Make sure your hands are under your shoulders.

- If push-ups on your knees are too difficult, do them standing up with your hands against a wall or a high surface such as a kitchen worktop (see page 129).

- Keep your elbows tucked into your side as you lower yourself down towards the floor.

- Return up to the starting position.

- Feel free to put a cushion or rolled-up blanket under your knees to protect them against the floor.

As in Simple Sweat (see page 143), feel free to choose one of the above five Easy Kneesy movements that you enjoy and repeat it over and over again in the prescribed time intervals, on page 135.

THE HIIT SQUAD

Challenge yourself with this advanced HIIT workout.

This is an advanced workout for people who are already pretty fit or have been doing the other Sweat health snacks and feel ready for a bigger challenge. If that sounds like you, you can join the HIIT Squad by completing this sequence of four exercises on every one of your Feel Better Days.

BURPEES

SHOULDER TAPS

SQUAT JUMPS

MOUNTAIN CLIMBERS

Do each exercise in sequence for one minute at full intensity, then rest for fifteen seconds in between each one.

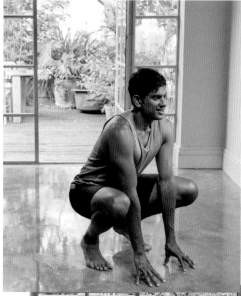

BURPEES

- From a standing position, drop down into a squat with your hands on the ground just in front of your feet.

- Kick your feet out behind you, keeping your arms straight so that you end up at the starting push-up position.

- Jump your feet back towards your hands and return to a squat position.

- Return to standing by jumping up in the air while raising your arms above your head.

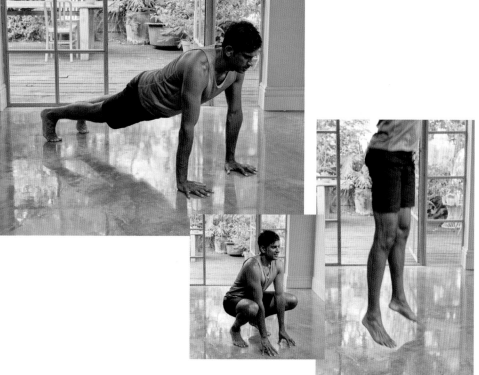

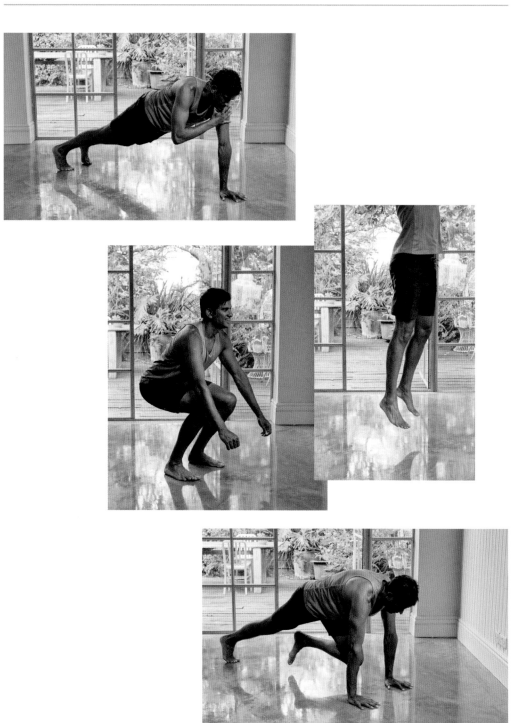

SHOULDER TAPS

- Position yourself as if you are about to start a push-up. From there, bring your right hand up to touch your left shoulder.

- Return your right hand to the floor and then bring your left hand up to touch your right shoulder.

- Alternate between the two sides as quickly as possible, making sure your core and glutes are tight and engaged throughout the entire movement. You'll know you're doing this because your body will remain fairly static and stable and the only thing moving will be your arms.

SQUAT JUMPS

- Start in a squat position with your feet shoulder width apart, and your thighs parallel to the ground. Your knees should be in line with your toes and your chest upright.

- From this position, jump as high as you can, raising your arms into the air at the same time.

- Try to land back in your squat position as softly as possible.

MOUNTAIN CLIMBERS

- Place yourself in a traditional push-up position, on your palms and toes. Your hands should be directly under your shoulders and you should feel as if your pelvis is being tucked under your body so the arch in your lower back disappears.

- Bring your right foot off the ground and bring the right knee forward under your chest.

- Return your right foot to the push-up position and switch legs.

- Continue, quickly alternating between legs: this is a fast movement.

This intense, advanced workout is almost impossible to do for more than five minutes but is superb for your cardiovascular fitness!

PLAY

It's only since I've become a father that I've realized just how unstoppably active children are. From the moment they first learn to crawl, it's as if they can't keep themselves still. Kids take such a simple, delightful pleasure in moving their limbs, interacting with balls and toys and tearing around as fast as they can on bikes and sleds and their own two feet. As we get older, for whatever reason, we seem to lose touch with this. Moving our bodies in any significant way comes to feel like a chore.

But this pleasure in movement and wearing ourselves out isn't the only thing we lose. Part of the primal joy in watching happy children at play is in seeing how they become utterly lost in what they're doing. Kids get so absorbed in the worlds of movement and fun they're creating that the rest of the world seems to just disappear. What this tells me is that the state we call being "mindful" and often work so hard to achieve is actually completely natural and normal. Before the pressures and responsibilities of adulthood kick in, we're able to access mindful states incredibly easily through play.

The following snack items involve reconnecting to this childhood state. I want you to throw off some of the self-importance and self-consciousness that tend to come with adulthood and just have some simple, silly, energetic fun.

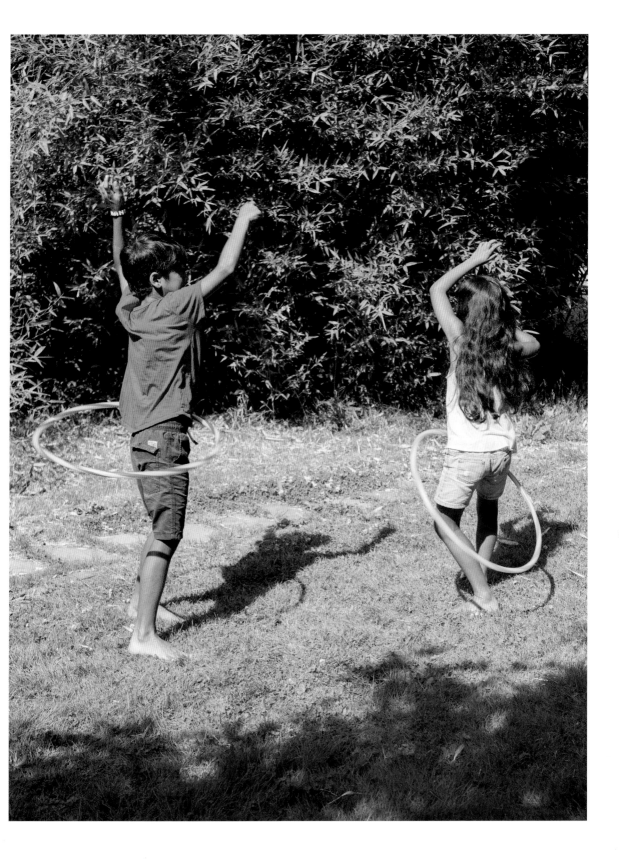

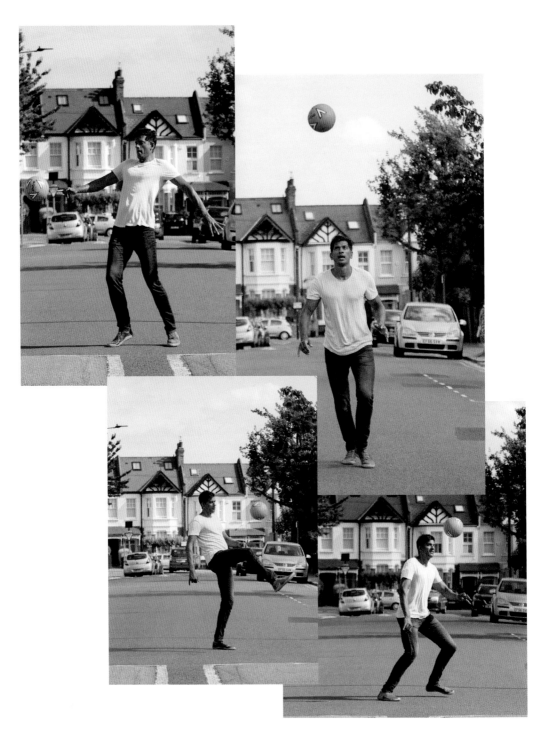

JUST PLAY!

Do some fun movements that make you feel like a child.

This is one of my favorite Play health snacks because it makes me feel so free and joyful. It's simple and unstructured and involves you just horsing around in constant motion.

Here are some of my favorite "Just Play!" movements:

- Play tag with your kids, grandkids, or friends in the backyard or around the house.

- Play basketball in the park or with a net in your backyard.

- Kick a ball around.

- Stand on a balance board in the living room.

Remember, these are simply some of my suggestions. Use them as a guide but feel free to come up with your very own Just Play! activities.

 You can listen to a fun conversation on my *Feel Better, Live More* podcast about the importance of play at drchatterjee.com/darryledwards

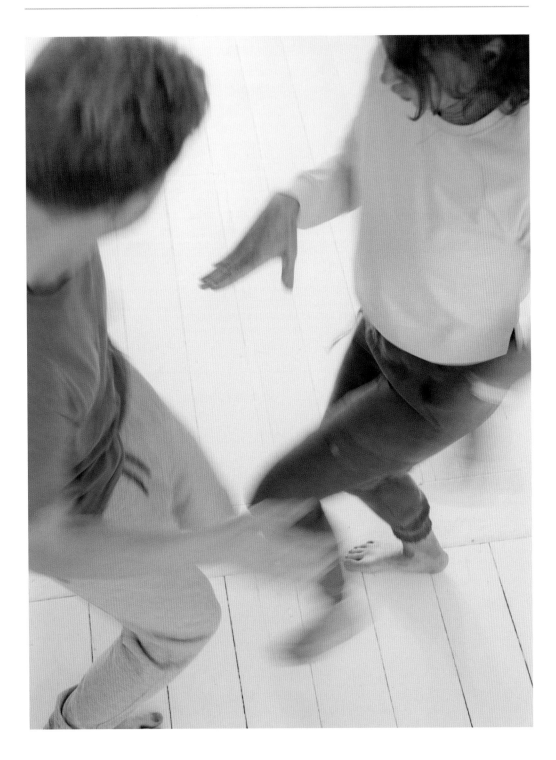

DANCING

Dance to a tune that makes you feel good.

Dancing is one of the most underrated ways to work out and get your heart pumping. You don't need to go to a class or wait until your next big night out with your mates. It's free and available to each and every one of us on a daily basis. Gym and Zumba instructors know all too well that music helps to motivate and keep people going, but you don't need to pay professionals to exploit this ancient and joyful activity.

I'd like you to simply choose an upbeat tune that inspires you and makes you feel good and just dance along, in whatever way you wish, for five minutes. Either set the song to repeat or choose a couple of high-tempo tracks and play them back to back. After five minutes of letting yourself leap about, your mood will have lifted, your energy levels will have risen and you'll feel much more motivated to do whatever else you have planned for the day.

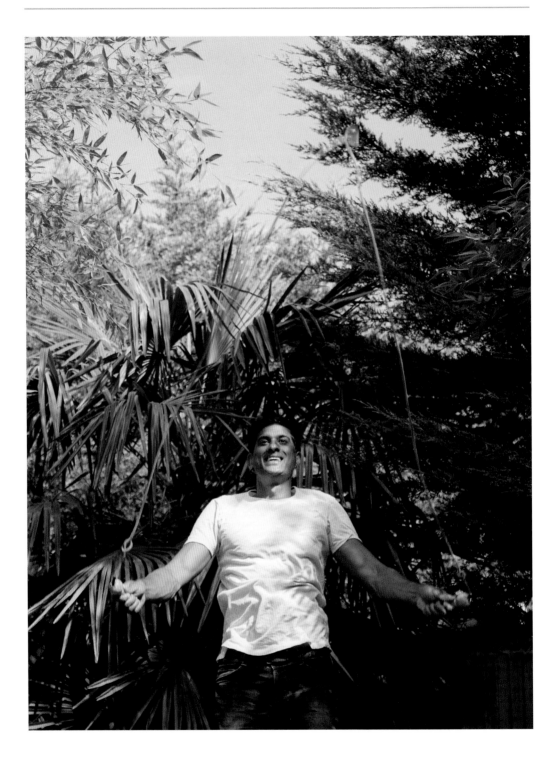

JUMPING ROPE

Dig out your rope and jump!

Jumping rope is one of the best ways to work out in a short period of time and helps with agility, balance, and coordination as well as cardiorespiratory fitness. It's best to start simple and then, as you become fitter and more confident, add in some more complex movements, such as:

- Criss-crossing arms

- Double hops

- Double unders

- High knees

- Jumping jacks

- Single legs

There are plenty of videos to watch on YouTube to give you more ideas as you become more skilled.

If you enjoy jumping rope, you can always incorporate it into the Simple Sweat workout. For example, thirty seconds of jumping followed by thirty seconds of rest five times will give you a brilliant five-minute workout that will be fun and leave you energized.

You can even do a mixture of all the Play health snacks mentioned in this section. For example, you could do one minute of jumping rope, one minute on a balance board and three minutes of dance. There are no rules—this is simply about five minutes of fun!

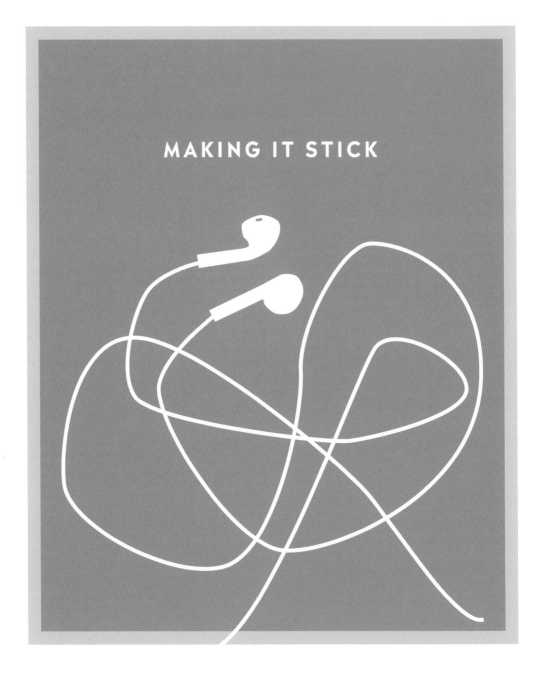

MAKING IT STICK

If you want to make any new behavior stick in the long term, it's really important to set up your environment so that engaging in your chosen behavior is as easy as possible.

Here are some tips that you may find helpful:

- Set up a playlist on your phone with your favorite feel-good tunes so you always have music ready to go to when it's time to dance.

- Make sure your jump rope is out somewhere visible. If you leave it in a cupboard, it is much less likely that you will use it.

- Keep your balance board out in the living room, bedroom, or kitchen, so that you are constantly being reminded that it is there.

- Keep the soccer ball in the middle of the backyard so that you see it every time you look out.

As you know by now, it is extremely helpful to stick your Play health snack on to an existing part of your daily routine. Why not do your 5 minutes of dancing every single evening right before you eat dinner? Or, what about leaving your jump rope by the front door and every day when you come in from work, it will act as a reminder to do your 5 minutes of jumping rope as soon as you get in?

CASE STUDY

It was the height of the scorching summer of 2018 and I could see how uncomfortable the heat was making Letitia. She was a forty-eight-year-old single mother who'd always struggled with her weight. She'd tried the gym and various workout classes but was concerned that people would stare at her because of her size. That day, Letitia had come in with her daughter, who was also overweight, and who she was worried about. Sixteen-year-old Namono seemed quite low and moody. At one point, she snapped at her mom, saying, "Well, you never go out either. You're just in the kitchen all day, listening to music." I got the strong impression that there were difficulties in their relationship.

But that wasn't what Letitia had come to see me about. I wondered if music might be the key to begin solving their worries around weight. Letitia always seemed to be wearing a Lady Gaga T-shirt and her daughter had a pair of headphones hanging off her neck. I mentioned that they both appeared to be music fans and that dancing can be a great way of exercising. I asked them to both choose one song of their choice, up tempo, and dance to it.

When they first started doing it, neither of them could get to the end of the five or six minutes of the song without stopping for breath. But after two weeks Namono could, and her mom, feeling competitive, soon caught her up. They were both thrilled to experience themselves becoming fitter in such a short time. It was a classic small victory.

But it's also had a brilliant Ripple Effect (page 25). It gave Letitia the confidence to start the "Couch to 5K" running program and motivated her to begin to change her diet. Not only are they both now losing weight, Namono has recently decided to join her mom on her running journey. They're fitter and healthier than they have been for years, and their tricky relationship has been transformed. And it all started with just five minutes of dancing.

BALANCE

Nature designed us to thrive in simpler times. We used to eat more simply, live more simply, and move around a lot more. Humans evolved to be physical creatures, hunting game, picking nuts and berries, building weapons, and gathering logs and leaves to make shelters.

But today we operate in a technological world in which so much of our physical labor has been replaced by psychological labor. Whether you're a teacher marking books, a retail assistant spending eight hours a day behind a high-tech checkout, an accountant bending towards your computer screen, a professional driver crouched over the steering wheel of your taxi or truck, or a studying student, a significant amount of your daily work is not muscle-based but brain-based.

This is a massive shift in how we are all spending our daily lives. And it's having a terrible effect on our posture. As we bend our busy brains towards our modern forms of work—and our televisions, tablets, and phones when we're not at work—we're changing the ways that our bodies function. For some of us, standing up straight with good posture can feel unnatural. For others, sitting up straight can be a real effort. Modern sedentary living is weakening all kinds of different muscles that are designed to support our skeleton. This can cause a whole host of problems, including back pain, shoulder pain and headaches.

One hugely important set of muscles that is woefully underused for many of us is our bottom muscles, or glutes. Our glutes are a keystone muscle, which means they're such a crucial part of our muscle network that, if we allow them to weaken through inactivity, it can have a negative effect on other parts of our body, from the shoulders right down to the feet.

But it's not just our glutes. Many important muscles, such as the ones that control our shoulder blades and our deep abdominal muscles (also known as our core), don't work as efficiently as they should and often stay switched off when they should be switched on. And because they are not doing the job they are supposed to be doing, our bodies start to compensate. Other muscles in the body try to take up the slack, but this comes at a cost. It's often not long before that has a knock-on effect and some muscles start to overwork, joints become overused and, before you know it, a little niggle turns into chronic, debilitating pain. Just as problematic is the fact that, if you don't use certain muscles or put your joints through their full range of motion, your body becomes less efficient and deskilled at performing certain basic movements. This is often the reason behind those classic cases of people bending over to pick up a pen and putting their back out.

The following two Balance health snacks have been designed to wake up your sleepy muscles and allow your body to experience the full range of movement that it's being starved of in our modern lives. They've been created in collaboration with Gary Ward (@garyward_aim), one of the world's leading thinkers on human movement.

You can listen to my *Feel Better, Live More* podcast to learn more about the importance of these Balance health snacks. Here are some great episodes to start with: drchatterjee.com/71 | drchatterjee.com/39 | drchatterjee.com/12

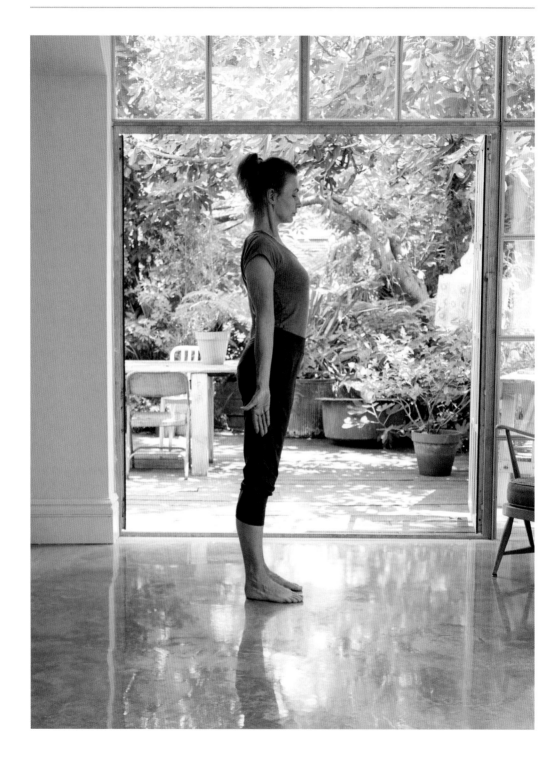

DESK JOCKEY WORKOUT

Spend five minutes undoing the damage of sitting down all day.

This health snack is particularly good if you spend most of your day sitting down, perhaps looking at screens. It can be incredibly helpful for back pain, neck pain, shoulder discomfort, and stiffness. It involves doing the following four exercises in sequence in the order prescribed.

WALL COGS

FRONTAL COGS

ARM SPIRALS

THE CRUCIFIX

Work through the above four exercises in sequence and then repeat. This will take you approximately five minutes.

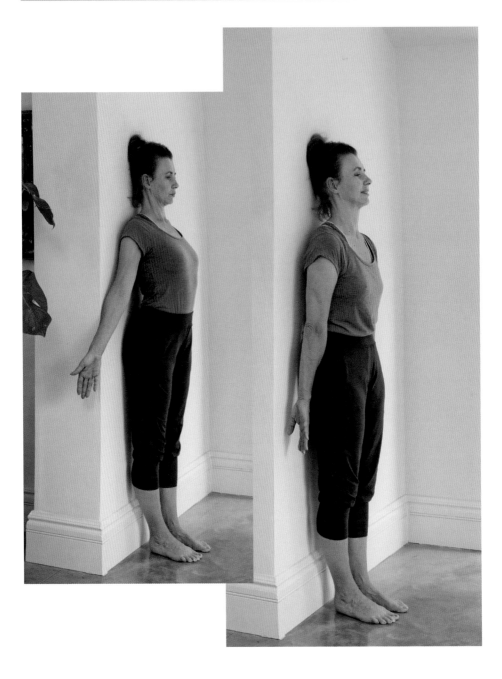

WALL COGS

This exercise will open up and mobilize your shoulder blades, spine, pelvis, and ribcage.

- Stand with your back to the wall. The back of your head, your shoulders, and your bottom should be touching the wall and your feet should be two to three inches away from it. Your arms should hang down naturally, palms facing in.

- For the duration of this exercise, ensure that there are always three points of contact with the wall: your bottom, your upper back and the back of your head.

- **Picture on left** Slide the back of your head up the wall. As you do this, you will feel your chin coming towards your chest a little. At the same time, feel as though your ribcage is lifting up and your chest is expanding. Imagine you are wearing a belt and the buckle is pointing towards the floor as the arch in your lower back gets bigger.

- As you're doing this, twist your hands outward, so that your palms face outwards and your thumbs point behind you. This will help to open up your shoulders and bring your shoulder blades towards each other, encouraging a full range of motion.

- **Picture on right** Now do the reverse. Slide your head back down the wall, past your starting position, until your eyes are looking up a little. At the same time, bring your ribcage down. Try to close the gap between your lower back and the wall so they become flush. As you do this, your imaginary belt buckle will start to point towards the ceiling. Your hands and arms will turn inwards, like a corkscrew.

- Move in and out of both positions. Repeat the above sequence ten times, while focusing on smooth and controlled movements. Quality is much more important than quantity, so stop as soon as you feel your form worsening.

To watch a video of this move, go to drchatterjee.com/wallcogs

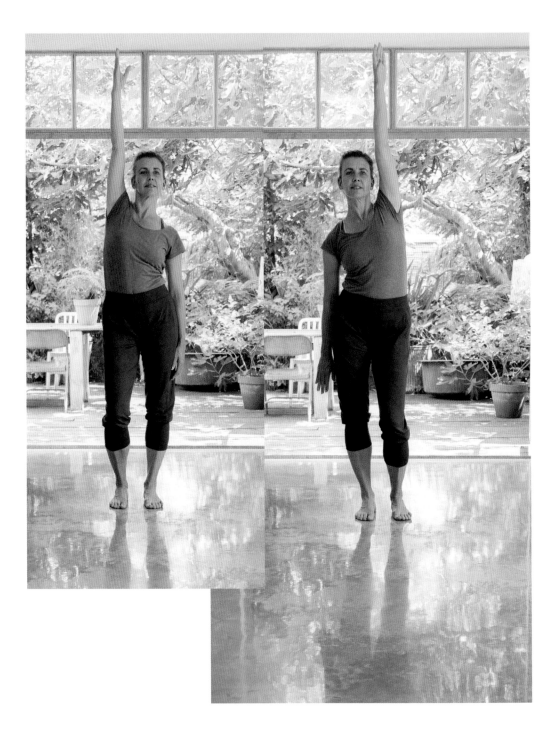

FRONTAL COGS

Frontal cogs are similar to wall cogs but work your body in a different plane. In this workout, you will use your back and chest muscles as well as your ribs.

- Stand up tall and straight.

- Bend your right knee forward while keeping both feet on the floor. As you do, feel the weight going into your left hip. Your left hip will hitch up and now be higher than your right hip.

- As you do this, reach your right arm up towards the ceiling. Really push it as high as it can go—**a common mistake is not to reach high enough!**

- Now do the reverse. Bend the left knee forward as the right knee straightens. Your right hip will now be higher than your left. Reach your left arm up as high as it will go. It is the reach that is most important here. **Think about reaching all the way into your fingertips**.

- Move in and out of both positions. Repeat the above sequence ten times, while focusing on smooth and controlled movements. Quality is much more important than quantity, so stop as soon as you feel your form worsening.

To watch a video of this move, go to drchatterjee.com/frontalcogs

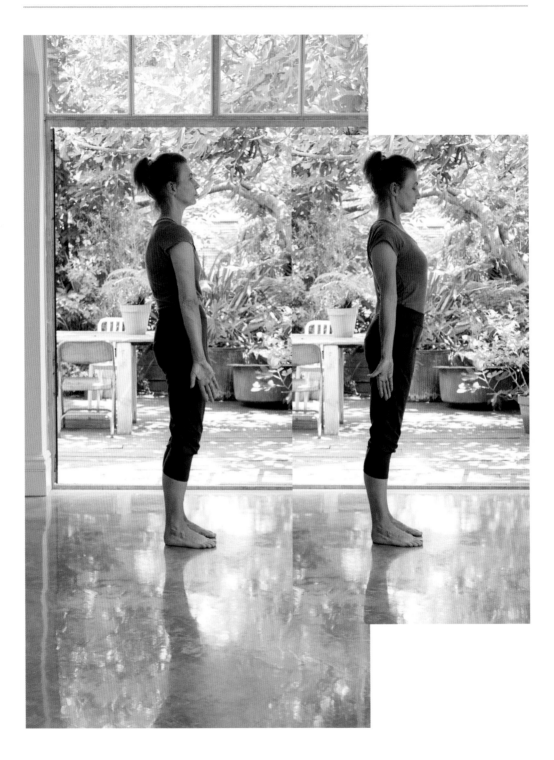

ARM SPIRALS

Our arms and shoulder blades are often chronically underused, especially in people who are stuck in chairs all day with their arms relatively immobile. This can lead to pain in our necks and shoulders and, sometimes, contribute to headaches. Arm spirals are a brilliant way to wake up your arms and shoulder blades and get them moving.

- Stand upright with both arms hanging by your sides in a relaxed manner. Your thumbs should be pointing out in front of you.

- **Picture on left** Turn your thumbs inwards as far as they will go so that they are pointing at the wall behind you. Your arms will feel like corkscrews as you do this movement and you will notice your shoulders rounding.

- **Picture on right** Now do the opposite. Turn out both your hands, arms and elbows as far as they'll go. Your thumbs will go full circle by coming round to point at the wall in front of you and then continuing until they point behind you. You should feel as if you're standing up nice and tall. Your shoulder blades should be squeezed together and your ribs and chest will be upright and open.

- Move in and out of both positions. Repeat the above sequence ten times, while focusing on smooth and controlled movements. Quality is much more important than quantity, so stop as soon as you feel your form worsening.

To watch a video of this move, go to drchatterjee.com/armspirals

THE CRUCIFIX

I've been doing the crucifix most days for years and it's helped enormously with my back pain and my posture. The beauty of this exercise is that it can be done anywhere, with no equipment, and it doesn't even get you sweaty.

- Stand up tall and straight with your arms in a "T" position. Your thumbs should be pointing straight out in front of you.

- **Picture on left** Turn your left arm fully inwards by bringing your left thumb down so that it starts to point to the floor and ends up pointing behind you. At the same time, turn your right arm fully outwards so that your right thumb starts to point towards the ceiling and ends up pointing behind you.

- Your left shoulder should become fully rounded so that, if you were to look over your left shoulder, you'd be able to see the top of your left shoulder blade.

- **Picture on right** From here, go to the opposite movement, with your right arm turning fully inwards and your left arm fully outwards.

- While performing each movement, try to keep your head level and feel as though your right and left arms are reaching out as far as possible, as if you're trying your best to pull your shoulder blades apart.

- Move in and out of both positions. Repeat the above sequence ten times, while focusing on smooth and controlled movements. Quality is much more important than quantity, so stop as soon as you feel your form worsening.

To watch a video of this move, go to drchatterjee.com/crucifix

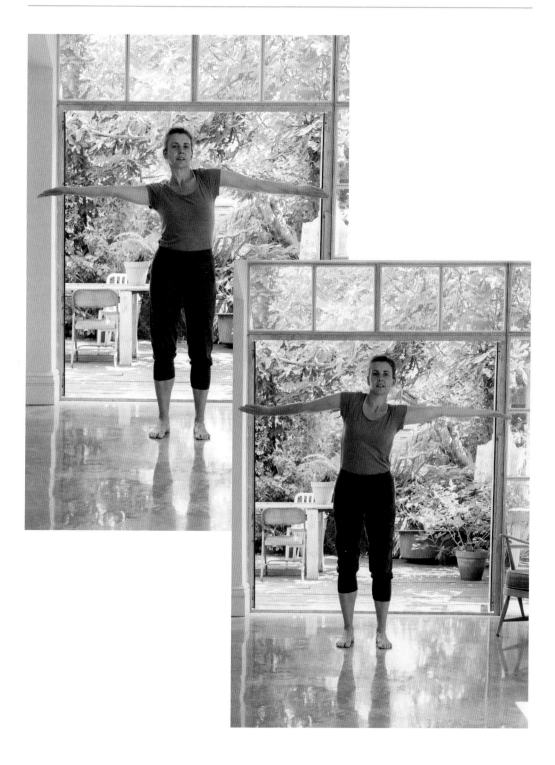

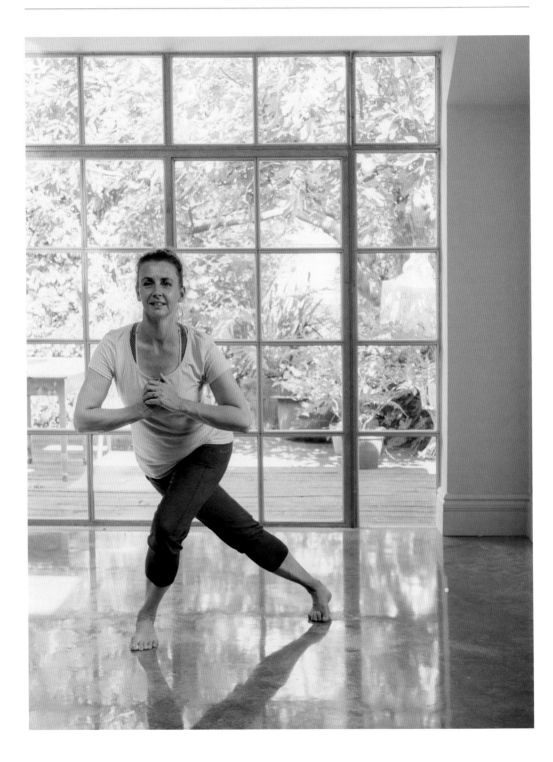

THE CLOCK WORKOUT

Wake up your body by moving it in all directions.

Much of our lives are spent moving our bodies in only one direction. Whether we're sitting on a chair, flexing our neck up and down to look at screens or moving between floors by going up and down stairs, we're drastically limited in our range of motions. Our bodies were designed to move in three dimensions, yet modern life forces us to largely move in only one.

This can contribute to pain and stiffness all over our body. Over the years, our bodies change and adapt to the lives that we have led, the injuries we have experienced and the repetitive behaviors we have employed. Certain muscles get overused while others don't get used enough. This can result in us experiencing problems when we try to be active. For example, some of us can no longer walk or run with optimal form, which can result in us experiencing pain or getting injured.

This clock workout is especially good for those of us who like to be active but spend a lot of time during the day sitting down. It can certainly help improve shoulder problems, elbow pain, hip stiffness, and back discomfort. But it's also a brilliant workout for prepping your body for your life when not sitting down. I often do it before I go for a run or swim.

LUNGE CLOCK

SHOULDER CLOCK

CORE CLOCK

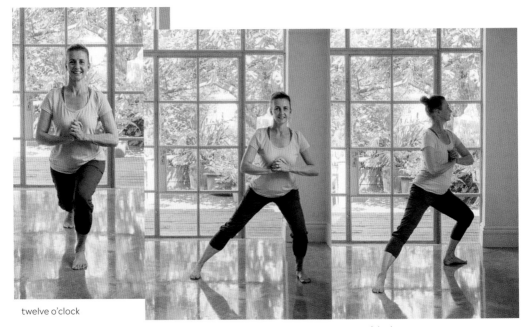

twelve o'clock

nine o'clock

seven o'clock

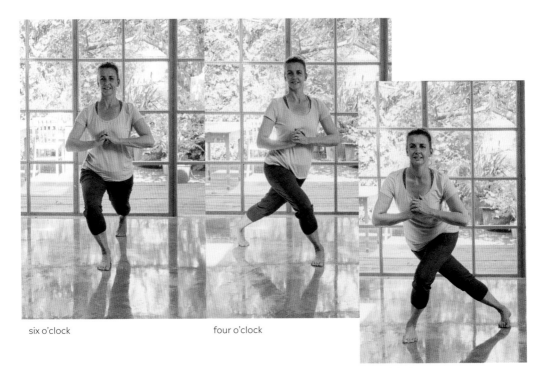

six o'clock

four o'clock

two o'clock

LUNGE CLOCK

This exercise will get your glutes working in every possible direction. Many cases of back pain have weak glutes as a contributory factor. The lunge clock is particularly beneficial for those who feel stiffness and pain in their lower back or who sit down all day at work. It will improve your strength, which will help you go up stairs more efficiently, run faster, and walk better. My approach prioritizes functionality over looks, but the simple fact is that when your bottom muscles are firing more efficiently, their shape will almost always improve.

- Stand with both your feet together.

- Lunge out towards twelve o'clock on an imaginary clock face with the left leg. Try to feel as if your weight is in the front of your left foot. Allow your body to go where it wants to go. It is perfectly OK for your knee to go past your ankle in this exercise, as this encourages full mobility in the feet.

- Bring the left leg back to the starting position.

- Lunge out to eleven o'clock with your left foot then return to the starting position. As you lunge, ensure that your right foot is still facing forward.

- Continue doing this sequence all the way round the clock.

- When you get to nine o'clock you will feel as though you are doing a sideways lunge (see photo).

- Lunging to six o'clock will feel like a reverse lunge, as most of your weight will be on your right foot. This will be the same for five o'clock, four o'clock and three o'clock.

- When you get to two o'clock, the left leg will again start to take most of the weight as it comes round and over (see photo).

- Repeat with the other leg. To do both sides will take approximately 90 seconds.

As you get better at doing the clock motions, you can make them more interesting, and challenging, by holding weights, water bottles, or cans of beans in each hand.

To watch a video of this move, as well as some tips on making them even more beneficial, go to drchatterjee.com/lungeclocks

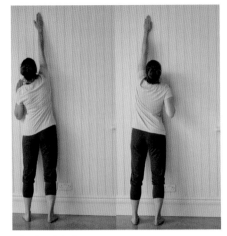

twelve o'clock

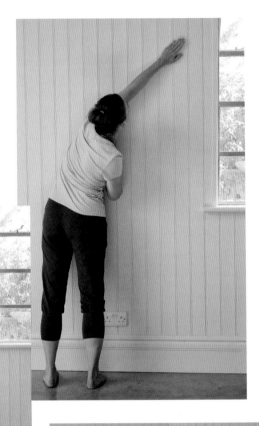

one o'clock

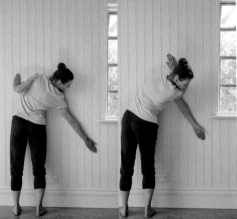

four o'clock

SHOULDER CLOCK

This exercise helps you to free up your upper back and shoulders from the prison of sedentary life. It can help if you suffer from shoulder or neck pain and stiffness. It can also help ease headaches.

The first time I did this exercise I felt as though my shoulder blades were being moved into positions they had never been in before. It felt fantastic.

- Stand facing a wall, about 12 inches away from it.

- Rest your bent forearms against the wall, out in front of your chest.

- Maintaining arm contact with the wall, reach up with your right hand to twelve o'clock. **Reach as far as you can**. The more you reach, the more movement you're exposing your shoulder joints and muscles to.

- Allow your body to follow your arm. Don't try to keep your body still— allow it to move in a way that enables you to reach your arm as far as possible along the clock point.

- Bring your right hand back to the starting position.

- Reach out with your left hand to twelve o'clock as far as you can, then bring your left hand back to the starting position.

- Now reach your right hand to one o'clock, and back.

- Repeat with the left hand.

- Continue this sequence, alternating hands around the whole clock face.

- When you are reaching with your left hand, say, to four o'clock, feel free to use the back of your hand rather than the palm (see photo).

- To go around the entire clock face will take approximately 90 seconds.

To watch a video of this move, go to drchatterjee.com/shoulderclocks

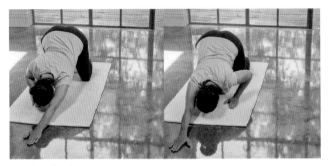

twelve o'clock

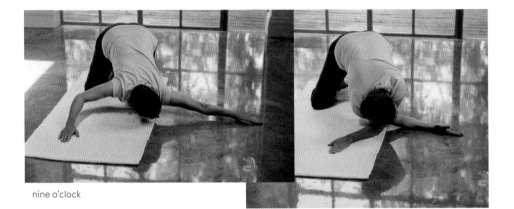

nine o'clock

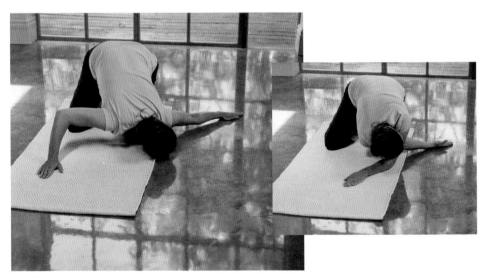

eight o'clock

CORE CLOCK

This exercise moves your whole body in a variety of different directions. It strengthens and mobilizes your abdominals, back, shoulder muscles, and spine. It is a brilliant whole-body movement that can be really helpful if you have pain and stiffness in your body at the end of a busy working day or as a great warm-up before you do something more active, such as going for a bike ride, a walk, or a run.

- Start off on all fours, with your knees under your hips and your hands under your shoulders. Slide your left hand out as far as possible in front of you to the twelve o'clock position.

- Reach as far as possible with your left hand and allow your body to follow. You will need to bend your right elbow to allow yourself to reach further. If your hips want to go out to the side to allow you to do this, great—don't stop them.

- Bring the left hand back to the starting position and repeat with the right hand. **Remember to reach out as far as you can.**

- Bring the right hand back to the starting position and then reach the left hand out as far as you can to eleven o'clock, then back. Repeat with the right hand.

- Keep going, around as many of the clock-face positions as you can, alternating from left to right hand.

- As you start to reach the side of the clock-face, you will sometimes need to use the back of your hands to reach. For example, when reaching out to nine o'clock (as in the photo opposite), your left hand will reach out with the palm facing down and your right hand will reach out with the palm facing up. **Remember to reach your hand as far as you can.**

- Once you have gone around as many clock positions as you can, return to the starting position.

- To go around the entire clock face will take approximately 90 seconds.

As you get stronger, you will soon be able to do this clock workout with your knees off the floor, in the starting position of a plank (forearms on the floor). To make the movement even more challenging, you can start off in a push-up position. With one arm supporting you, reach out the other to as many of the clock-face numbers as possible.

To watch a video of this move, go to drchatterjee.com/coreclocks

CASE STUDY

Ian was one of those patients who don't really come to the doctor's much, even when they are poorly. He worked at a help desk for a transport company and he told me that over the last few months he'd been suffering from lower-back pain and that it would get progressively worse as the day went on. By the end of his shift, he'd often also feel a little niggle at the base of his neck on the right-hand side. He'd asked for a standing desk but had been denied permission by his boss. He'd been treating himself with strong over-the-counter painkillers. He came to see me when the pain began interfering with his Saturday park-run sessions, which were the one thing he'd look forward to all week.

When I saw Ian, there was a six-week wait in our practice for a physical therapist. During this period, I gave him the Desk Jockey Workout to do. I told him there were multiple things that could be contributing to his pain, including bending over a screen and being on the phone all day. Our body is designed to move with a whole different range of motions, but our jobs often restrict us to one plane or dimension of movement. I told Ian that this particular workout would remind his entire body of all the different movements that it was regularly neglecting.

Within days, Ian found that his back was a bit looser and the niggles in his neck started to reduce in strength and frequency. By the time I saw him two weeks later, his neck pain had gone completely. "My back is still pretty bad," he said, "but it certainly feels a lot looser after I've done the exercise."

Because he'd felt the difference the Desk Jockey Workout could make for him, he promised to start doing it at work as well. As soon as it hit one o'clock he'd go to a storage room that didn't get used much and spend five minutes doing the workout. Three weeks later I got a message to say that Ian had canceled his appointment with the phyiscal therapist.

RESTORE

After long hours spent tearing around from place to place, when we've finally got some time to ourselves what we often need is some movement that will settle us, ground us, and restore us. If we choose the right form of activity we can turn these five minutes into one of the most special and relaxing parts of our day.

For me, that means yoga. This is a practice that began over five thousand years ago, which makes it older than the Pyramids. It constantly blows my mind that I can have a direct connection with such an ancient people on an average rainy day in South Manchester, simply by slowing down, breathing, and stretching myself into some basic yogic postures, some of which can still be seen on precious time-worn wall carvings in northern India.

I completely understand if you have reservations about yoga. Countless patients of mine say it's not their cup of tea, but, almost always, I've managed to change their minds. I'd encourage you to put aside your pre-existing ideas and trust me. The chances are, you'll like it.

Modern science has only just begun catching up with what the ancients seemed to intuitively know—that yoga is great for us, body and soul. Over the last few years clinical research has found that yoga can reduce levels of stress and anxiety, help combat fatigue, is good for your heart, and helps

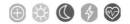

you sleep better. There's even evidence to suggest it can help alleviate serious psychological disorders, including depression and PTSD.

The reality is that yoga-based movements can be the perfect antidote to many of the stresses of the modern world. One of the things that makes yoga so effective is that it's an amazing combination of stretching, focus, and breathing. I love it because it's good for the whole system: mind, body, and heart. After a great yoga session you feel chilled and energized, which is not how you always feel after a hard session at the gym or a HIIT workout in your front room.

I've put together two simple yoga sequences, each of which should take no more than five minutes to complete.* You don't need to be an expert to do them. You don't even need a yoga mat, although many do like to practice with one. When you're working through these sequences, I'd like you to really focus on slowing down and enjoying some time to yourself.

*Of course, I have checked both sequences with a qualified yoga teacher.

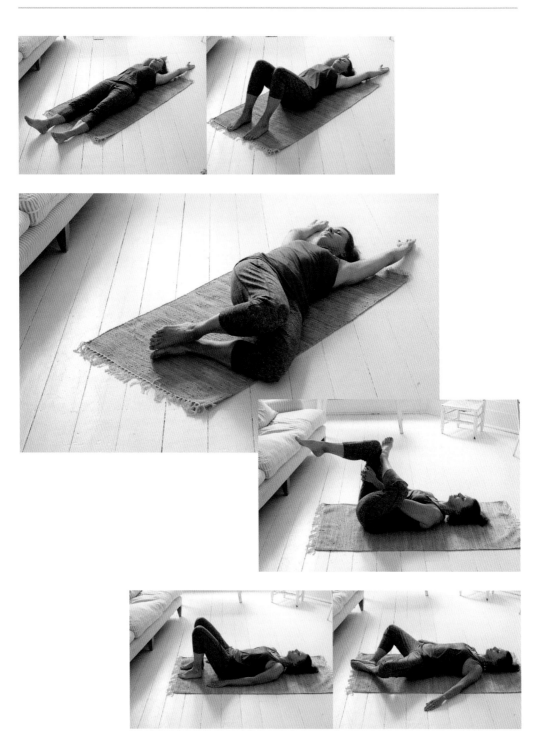

THE MORNING WAKE-UP FLOW

Wake up your body with this enjoyable, relaxing sequence.

This gentle sequence works especially well in the morning, helping your body to wake up. It's super-simple and amazingly relaxing. Stay in each position for five deep breaths, which takes thirty seconds or so. This way, you won't need to interrupt the flow by constantly checking your timer.

- Lie on your back with arms outstretched above your head. Take deep breaths for around thirty seconds—this is usually around five breaths.

- Slowly bend your knees so that your feet are flat on the floor.

- Keeping your back on the floor and your arms outstretched above your head, move your knees over to the left. Breathe in and out deeply five times. On each exhale see if you can sink further and further into the stretch.

- Repeat on the other side for five breaths.

- Bring your left foot on top of your right knee. Clasp your hands behind your right knee and gently pull it towards your chest. You'll feel a stretch in your left hip and glute.

- Take five deep breaths. With every out-breath try to sink a little further into the stretch.

- Repeat on the other side for five deep breaths.

- Bring your feet back to the floor. Keep your knees bent and your arms relaxed by your side.

- Allow both knees to fall outwards to the side, trying to keep your feet together. If this stretch feels too much, put some pillows under each knee to lessen it. Take five deep breaths in this position. On each exhale see if you can sink further and further into the stretch.

- Rise up from your lying position and sit down on your knees with your hips on your heels. If you need to, put a cushion between your hips and heels for comfort.

- Stretch both hands out in front of you, bringing your head to the floor. Take five deep breaths in this position.

- Rise up on to all fours with your shoulders directly over your wrists and your hips directly above your knees. Try to keep your back fairly straight and feel that your stomach muscles are gently tensed.

- Take a deep breath. As you exhale, arch your back, let your stomach muscles relax and allow your head and tailbone to go towards the sky.

- As you inhale, round your back, tuck your chin in towards your chest, and feel as if your tailbone is facing the ground.

- Move in and out of these two positions five times, remembering to inhale as you round your back and exhale as you arch it.

- On the final exhale bring your hips down to sit on top of your heels with both knees on the ground. Keep your upper body straight and upright.

- Take a deep breath. As you exhale, put your left hand behind you on the floor facing backwards—put it where it feels comfortable; it does not need to be flat on the floor.

- Bring your right hand to the outside of your left knee. Pull gently on your left knee and feel your chest turning outwards. You should feel a gentle stretch in your upper back. Hold for five deep breaths.

- Repeat on the opposite side.

- To finish, stretch both arms overhead, feeling your back arch as you do a slight backbend.

This movement sequence is a fantastic way to start your day and many people find that when they do it they feel more relaxed, calmer, and less anxious for the entire day. Not bad for just five minutes first thing in the morning!

Of course, this movement flow can also be done at other times. It's a great way to de-stress at the end of a busy work day or to unwind and relax just before bed to help promote deep, relaxing sleep.

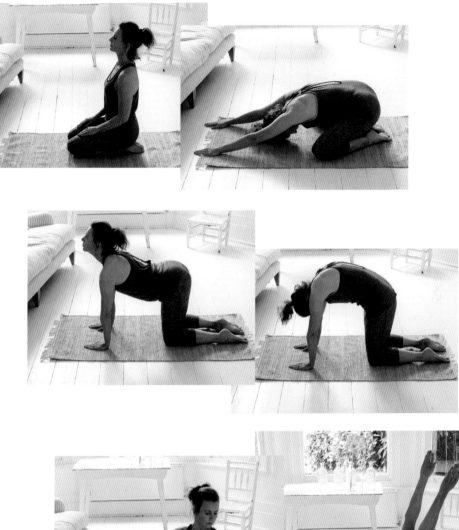

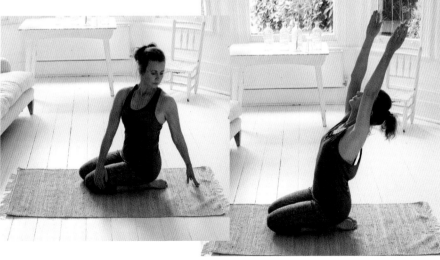

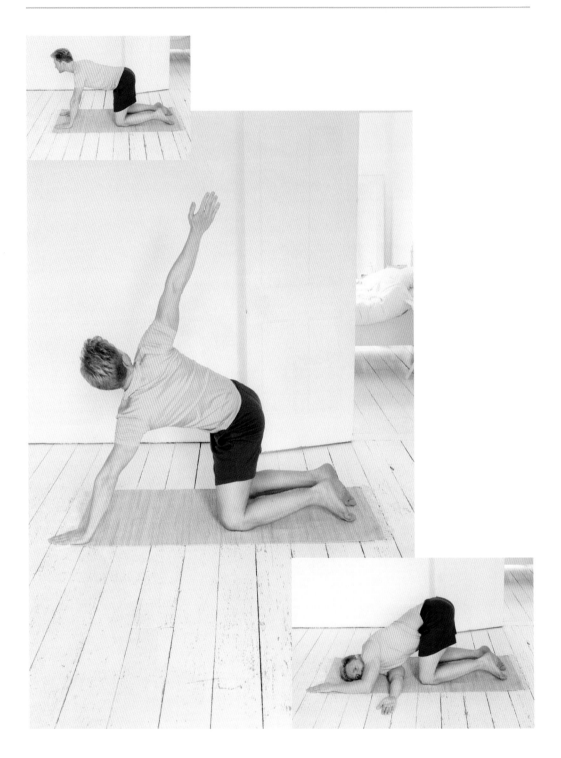

THE DAY'S END RELEASE FLOW

Enjoy some calm with these relaxing moves.

This five-minute unwind sequence will help loosen you up and is particularly good if you tend to feel tight in your back and shoulders after a long day. It should feel calming and won't leave you feeling out of breath. Don't get concerned if some of the moves feel tricky at first. Do what you can. The more you practice, the easier it will feel. The goal is to do each pose for roughly one minute.

THREAD THE NEEDLE

This pose will help open up your chest and work on relieving the tension that often builds up between your shoulder blades and in your back muscles after a long day in the office, a long commute, or running around after your kids.

- Start on all fours. Walk your hands forward a little so that they sit ahead of your shoulders.

- Pressing down through your left hand, breathe in and extend the right arm out and up towards the ceiling.

- As you exhale, slide your right hand under your left shoulder and stretch outwards as far as it will go. If you can, bring your right shoulder to the floor, bending the left elbow. Go as far as feels comfortable.

- Relax in this position and take five deep breaths. Every time you breathe out, try to deepen the stretch a little.

- On the final exhale, push through your left palm and replace your right hand alongside it, returning to the starting position.

- Repeat on the other side.

- Aim to do for thirty seconds on each side (around five deep breaths).

PUPPY-DOG STRETCH

This pose will help with tight shoulders and upper-back issues. If you're just starting out and want to make it easier, try resting your forehead on a pillow or a folded blanket. This will take some of the tension out of the stretch.

- Start on all fours, with your hips over your knees and your shoulders over your wrists.

- Keeping your back straight, extend your arms forward, keeping your hips above your knees. As you do, feel your forehead moving towards the floor. Don't worry if your forehead doesn't reach it—go as far as you feel comfortable. You should feel a relaxing stretch in your shoulders and upper back.

- If you're a little tight in your shoulders, move your hands outwards, as this will ease the stretch.

- Take deep breaths until your minute is up (around ten deep breaths).

THE ABDOMINAL STRETCH

This is not a classical yoga pose—I learned it from an osteopath friend who believes that everyone should be doing it every single day. The first time I tried it, it felt amazing. I was stretching muscles I'd never stretched before. It's great for toning your spine and helps to promote its natural curvature in those of us who spend a long time sitting at desks or behind a steering wheel.

- Start on all fours, with your hands beneath your shoulders and your knees beneath your hips.

- Turn both hands outwards so that your fingers are pointing away from your body and shuffle both knees back a little.

- Drop your hips as far as you can towards the ground and feel your back arching. You might have to play around a little to find the exact position you're looking for.

- Ideally, you want to feel a light stretching sensation throughout the front of your body, especially in your abdominal muscles.

- You can up the ante by lifting your head and gazing up towards the sky. Stay in this position, breathing naturally until your minute is up (around ten deep breaths).

- If you feel this stretch is putting strain on your back, stop and repeat one of the other exercises instead.

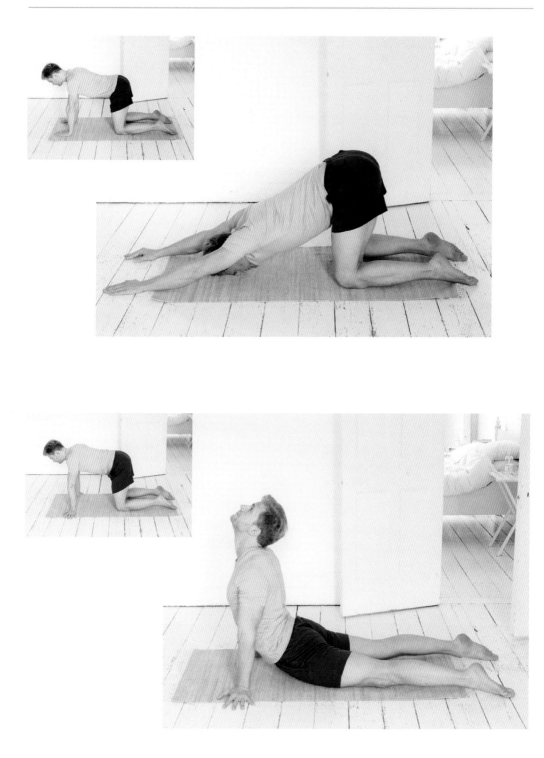

PIGEON POSE

This fantastic stretch really helps open up the hips and glutes. If you love it as much as I do, I would recommend going to a local yoga class to learn some of the more complex variations.

- Start on all fours, with your hands beneath your shoulders and your knees beneath your hips.

- Bring your right knee towards your right hand, then bring your right ankle as far as you comfortably can towards your left wrist.

- Extend your left leg outwards behind you, making sure your left knee and the front of your left foot are on the ground. If you need to, you can pop a cushion or a blanket underneath your knee.

- Try to make sure your hips are square to each other and facing forwards.

- Bend forward at the waist. As you do so, you will feel the stretch in your right glute start to deepen. Go as far as feels comfortable.

- If you want to alter the stretch, try to drape your chest over your front shin.

- In whichever position you find most comfortable, take five deep breaths (this will take about 30 seconds).

- To come out of the stretch, slowly walk your hands back towards you.

- Repeat on the other side.

Note: This can be a very intense pose and there are a number of variations you can try, depending on your current flexibility. If your hips are really tight, the angle of your front shin will probably point towards your opposite hip. That is fine. With time, the aim is to work towards bringing your front shin up and to get it as close as you can to being at right angles to your chest. It can feel quite challenging if you have never done it before. The more you practice it, the easier it will get.

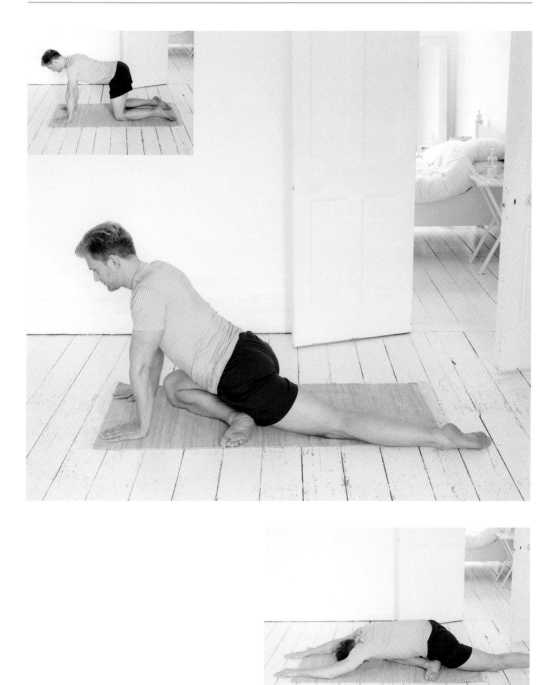

TRIANGLE POSE

This is a brilliant stretch that opens up parts of the body that are often neglected, like our sides, groin, and waist. It is a pose that most people are able to do and helps make you more body-aware.

- Stand, then step your right foot out to the side. Rotate your right foot out to 90 degrees to your chest and turn in your left foot slightly. You may find it easier to practice this pose with your back against the wall. This helps to maintain good posture throughout.

- Raise your arms to shoulder height and take a deep breath in.

- As you exhale, reach and extend your chest over your right leg, keeping it in line with your body, and allow your right hand to rest on your right shin.

- Extend your left arm up overhead, stretching through your fingertips. Try to stack your shoulders on top of one another and look up towards your left palm.

- You may need to alter the position of your right hand on your right shin to find the level of stretch that is comfortable for you. Don't place your right hand on your right knee as this can cause too much strain.

- Once in a comfortable position, take five deep breaths (this will take about thirty seconds).

- Repeat on the other side.

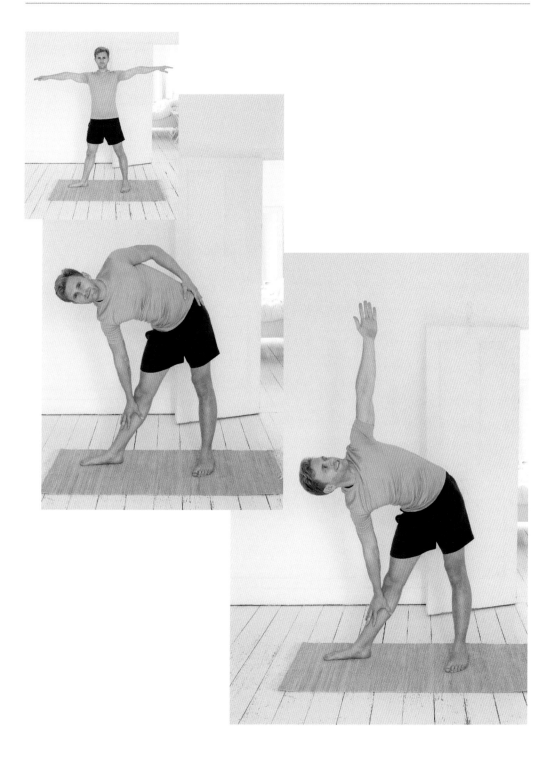

CASE STUDY

Brian used to love rugby, but one afternoon at a local match he sustained a serious knee injury that ultimately stopped him playing for good. His performance on the pitch had been of immense importance to his self-esteem and he rapidly became depressed. Matters worsened when the sudden drop in intense physical activity caused him to move less and snack on junk food and, as a result, put on weight. Brian began isolating himself and had come to my clinic with the expectation that I'd prescribe him an antidepressant.

Instead, I suggested yoga. The practice wouldn't put much pressure on his knees but he would still feel that he was being physically challenged. I thought that, as well as working on his body, it would also help his mind calm down and improve his focus. I suggested that Brian join a local yoga class so he could learn the correct movements from an instructor. He wasn't at all keen on this and looked embarrassed at the thought, so I decided to signpost him to a couple of YouTube yoga videos that I had previously used myself.

When I caught up with Brian a few weeks later I was encouraged to find that, when I asked how the yoga was going, his face visibly brightened. "I can't do a couple of these moves," he said. "I thought it would be easy. I've been really getting into it and joined a local class. I'm absolutely determined to crack these moves."

This was exactly the response I'd been hoping for. Brian was clearly experiencing that wonderful feeling of flow when he was doing his yoga. He was getting lost in the challenge. The pursuit of perfecting his moves seemed to be giving him back some of the purpose that had been missing from his life since his knee injury had taken him off the rugby pitch.

Even better, the Ripple Effect I'd hoped for had also appeared. Brian quickly realized that if he was going to get better at yoga more quickly he'd have to start looking after his diet. When he got in from work he used to treat himself to a packet of crisps or a glass of wine. Now he goes straight into his yoga session. He skipped the snack and had a wholesome but healthy evening meal earlier than he would have done before. Because the yoga made him feel so good he felt less of an urge to drink alcohol in the evening, which in turn helped him to sleep better. Within weeks, his mood had significantly improved.

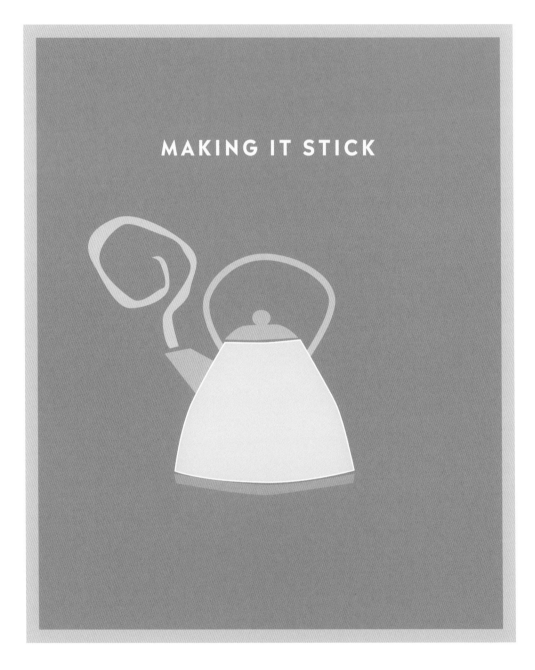

MAKING IT STICK

I know I've said this before, but I really cannot emphasize it enough. I would strongly recommend that you stick your Body health snack on to a regular part of your daily routine. This will make it much more likely that you will consistently be able to perform it. The following times work really well:

AS SOON AS YOU WAKE UP

IN THE KITCHEN WHILE MAKING A HOT DRINK

IMMEDIATELY BEFORE YOU EAT YOUR LUNCH

AS SOON AS YOU GET HOME FROM WORK

JUST BEFORE DINNER

Initially, I would recommend that you do the same Body health snack every day. This helps to remove decision fatigue. If you have to decide each time which specific health snack to do, it can lead to indecision, which starts off the procrastination process, which often leads to doing nothing at all. If you learn one of the workouts and repeat it day after day, you start to lock in that new behavior and it is rewarding to see your progress.

Having said that, once you have found a regular time to do your Body health snack and it is starting to become automatic, you can change it up, depending on how you feel. For example, you may usually perform a Strength workout as soon as you get home from work, but you might be exhausted and feel like doing a restorative yoga flow instead. As you progress in the *Feel Better in 5* program you will start to understand your body better and be able to personalize the program to your life.

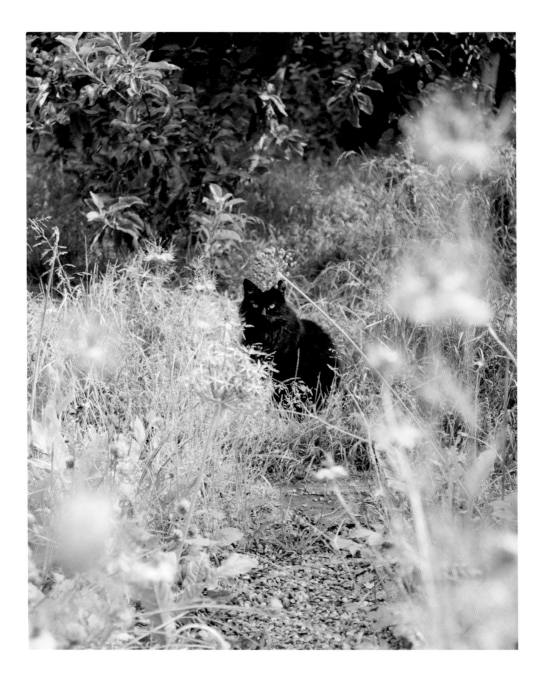

3
HEART

I STRONGLY BELIEVE THAT THE WORLD
WOULD BE A MUCH HEALTHIER PLACE IF WE ALL
SPENT A BIT MORE TIME STRENGTHENING OUR
BONDS WITH OTHERS

HEART SNACKS MENU

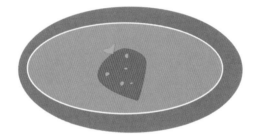

CHOOSE **ONE** HEALTH SNACK
TO **NOURISH YOUR HEART**

CONNECT

THE LOVE LIST | TEA RITUAL | THE KINDNESS PRACTICE

CALL A FRIEND | THE LOCAL CAFÉ

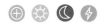

FORGIVE

THE FORGIVENESS PRACTICE | THE FORGIVENESS AFFIRMATION

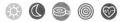

CELEBRATE

THE GRATITUDE GAME | GRATITUDE FOR LIFE

DAILY PLEASURE | CELEBRATE YOURSELF

CELEBRATE OTHERS | REFRAME THE MOMENT

REFRAME THE DAY | REFRAME THE FUTURE

HEART

What is happiness?

Does it come from buying fancy things? Fancy vacations? Fancy clothes? Expensive meals? Of course, all these things can be extremely pleasurable, and there's nothing wrong with enjoying them. But I don't believe pleasure and happiness add up to the same thing. For me, happiness is not a feeling that comes from the stomach, a wine bottle, or the wallet. It's not an exotic location you can get to on a long-haul fight. True happiness comes from our connections with other people. It comes from the heart.

Over almost twenty years of seeing patients I've learned that our hearts are one of the most important organs for our health. They're not just pumps that deliver oxygen around the body. They're also those slightly magical things that poets, storytellers, and songwriters have been waxing lyrical about for hundreds of years. Our hearts enable us to feel love, to connect with others, and to connect us to ourselves.

I fully appreciate that some of you may feel slightly skeptical about the importance of some of the health snacks in this section. However, I've seen time and time again that it's simply not possible to be truly happy and healthy if you feel disconnected from the people around you. And it's not just me who says so. Modern science is now starting to back up what all those romantic artists have been saying for so long.

It's only recently become clear how critical good connections are to our wellbeing. People who are lonely are 50 percent more likely to die earlier and 30 percent more likely to suffer from a heart attack or stroke. The feeling of social isolation is now thought to be as harmful to your health as smoking fifteen cigarettes a day. When you feel isolated, your body thinks it's under threat and vulnerable to attack because you don't have a supportive community around you to keep you safe. In order to protect you, it activates its stress response, which in turn ramps up your immune system. This triggers a process called inflammation. If this inflammation goes on for too long, it can contribute to the development of conditions such as type 2 diabetes, autoimmune conditions, strokes, and heart attacks.

This is why I've made maintenance of connections one of the three key pillars of the *Feel Better in 5* program. It's a hugely neglected part of both mental and physical wellbeing. I'd go as far as to say that while Mind and Body are critical aspects of health to address, this Heart section is arguably the most important area of them all to address. I strongly believe that the world would be a much healthier place if we all spent a bit more time strengthening our bonds with others. I love doing my Heart health snacks in the evening, as I find they're an amazing way of winding down and reminding myself what's really important after the stresses of a long day.

CONNECT

The deep power of connection.

To understand why connection is so crucial to health we first have to realize that we're a very peculiar kind of animal that has evolved to depend upon it in an unusually deep way. As a species, we're often compared to chimpanzees. These great apes might be our closest evolutionary cousins and behave like us in ways that can seem spookily similar. But we're unlike them in one extremely important way. Humans are incredibly cooperative. We work together. We rely on each other. We're designed to survive and thrive by being connected to one another. This is why we feel joyful and safe when we're getting along well with the people we share our lives with. We're wired to feel good when we connect because connection has always been critical to our survival. These wonderful positive emotions are nature's way of telling us we're successful members of the human species and that things are going well.

But the stresses and strains of modern life can do great damage to these connections. In our deep evolutionary pasts we had plenty of time to keep our close relationships oiled and healthy. We'd have spent time walking to the hunt and catching up with each other on the way. We'd have chatted to our neighbors as we picked berries and prepared food. Even as recently as ten years ago, we had precious minutes at the bus stop, in the supermarket queue or in the doctor's waiting room when we could chat to others.

Today, due to the extraordinary rise of smartphones, even those last scraps of opportunity to connect have largely disappeared. As a species, we've never been less connected. We go to church less, we join clubs less, we gather together in communities less. This can't be good for us. Human connection is as important as any vitamin or nutrient.

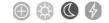

When was the last time you struck up a conversation with a stranger?

Or asked them how their day was going?

Or complimented them on their outfit or choice of book?

And this lack of connection is having a devastating impact on our closest relationships. It's a terribly sad fact that about 40 percent of US marriages currently end in divorce. While there are many different reasons for this, one of the most common sources I see among my patients is the simple fact that we're all too busy. The harsh realities of modern life mean that many of us are not prioritizing time with our partners. We live in a time in which both parents typically work, the extended family is not around so much to support us and we're continually being distracted by screens. Our relationships are under attack by our twenty-first-century lifestyles.

The following health snacks are all about improving the quality of our connections with friends, family, and partners. Just five minutes a day, on each of your Feel Better Days, spent nurturing these vital relationships can have a wonderful effect on your mood and your physical health.

FB
LM

To hear to an inspiring conversation about the power of connection and community listen to my *Feel Better, Live More* podcast on this topic at drchatterjee.com/happypear

THE LOVE LIST

Write down five things you love about someone close to you.

This health snack involves finding a quiet place where you can think about and write down five things you love about someone close to you. It could be your partner, child, a parent, a work colleague, your boss. You can choose a different person to write about each day or stick to the same person and write down more good things about them. When you go through the process of thinking about and then writing down the things you love about someone else, it can be deeply moving. When you write something down, the exercise tends to be more powerful, as the act of writing forces you to slow your mind a little and really process what you are thinking about.

Because humans are natural problem solvers we tend to automatically focus our attention on the negative aspects of the people we love. We might be annoyed that our partner always leaves the milk out on the counter, forgetting about all the other wonderful qualities they have. We might focus on irritating things, like one of your friends always having to choose where you go out to eat, at the same time forgetting what a good friend they are. By forcing ourselves to focus on the positive, even for five minutes, we can transform our relationships for the better.

Patients regularly report back to me that, by practicing this health snack regularly, they increase their focus and become happier, calmer, less resentful, and more patient. By looking at other people in a more compassionate frame of mind, they inevitably become better people themselves.

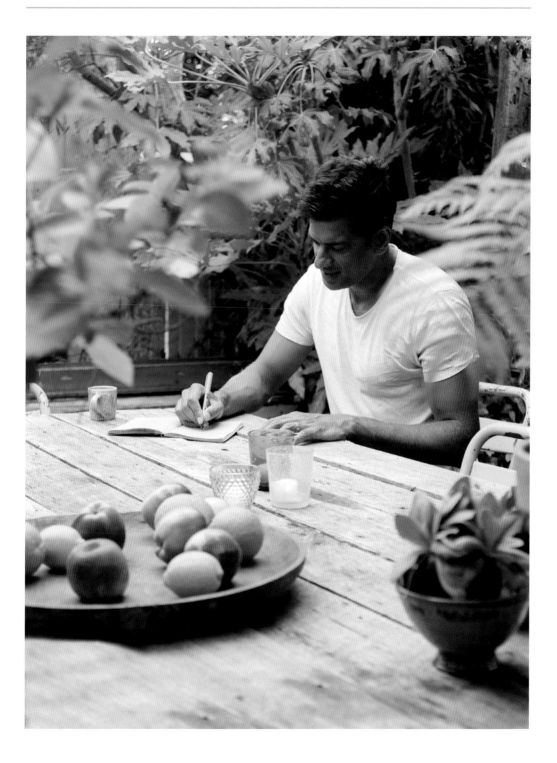

TEA RITUAL

Stop what you are doing and sit attentively with a friend or partner.

This health snack is about having five minutes each day in which you stop what you're doing and prioritize your relationships. This could be your relationship with a romantic partner but could just as easily be your relationship with a roommate or a friend. At a fixed time each day, perhaps in the evening after you've washed the dishes, rather than mindlessly putting on the television or rushing to finish some work, put the kettle on to boil, get a teapot, and make a cup of tea together. I'd recommend you go for something herbal, as anything with caffeine in it can have a negative impact on your sleep. Having a ritual around this time helps to make it into an event, which makes it feel more meaningful and precious.

Sit down with your partner or close friend in a calm and tidy place, without the TV on or any digital devices in view. Make eye contact. Sit attentively. Talk. Not about finances or who's taking the kids to their parties or clubs on the weekend. Find out about each other's day. Discover what's really going on in each other's life beyond the superficial distractions of everyday life. Try to listen attentively. Show that you are actively listening by nodding your head. Try not to interrupt when the other person is speaking and don't try to impose your own "solutions" to what the other person is saying. This health snack is not about solving problems, it is about listening and connecting.

Of course, you don't have to do this in the evening. One of my patients does this health snack during her lunch break each day. She'd come to see me complaining of low mood, indifference, and not really enjoying her job. She made a plan to spend five minutes every lunch break having a cup of tea in the staff café with a work colleague she felt close to. They made a vow not to talk about work during their break. Those five minutes of connection alone had an immediate effect on her wellbeing. Within days, she was feeling happier and more content both in and out of work. I hear this outcome a lot in my practice. Ultimately, this simple health snack feeds a critical part of your body that craves daily nourishment—your heart.

Listen to a conversation I have with the inspirational Johann Hari about the importance of meaningful human connection on my *Feel Better, Live More* podcast at drchatterjee.com/johannhari

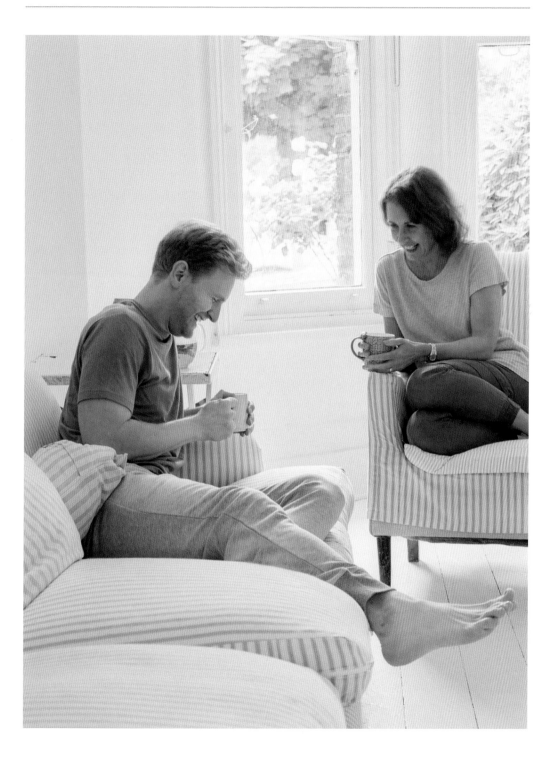

THE KINDNESS PRACTICE

Perform a five-minute act of kindness.

Recent research confirms that kindness can be incredibly beneficial for our wellbeing. Kindness can reduce pain, anxiety, and depression, and give you more energy, as well as make you happier and extend your life. One study from the Yale School of Medicine found that people who perform more acts of kindness in a day are more resilient to stress and have a more positive outlook on life.

This is why, for this health snack, I'd like you to spend up to five minutes performing a simple act of kindness. You could send one of your contacts in your phone a meaningful text telling them how much you value them or thanking them for something they've done, either recently or a long time ago. It could be a little note you write to your kids for when they wake up in the morning. You could pop by to say hello to an elderly neighbor on your way back home. You could strike up a conversation with the barista who made your latte and thank them for making it just the way you like it. There are infinite ways to do this, so be as imaginative as you can.

We are often so busy we don't let the people around us know how much we value them. Doing so is so easy, it doesn't have to cost anything, and we can give them a wonderful, warm glow that they can carry with them for the rest of the day. I often imagine how much happier the world would be if everyone in it did a small act of kindness every day. It would change everything.

FB
LM
You can listen to an inspiring conversation about the importance of kindness on my *Feel Better, Live More* podcast, when I spoke to the Buddhist monk Haemin Sunim, at drchatterjee.com/62

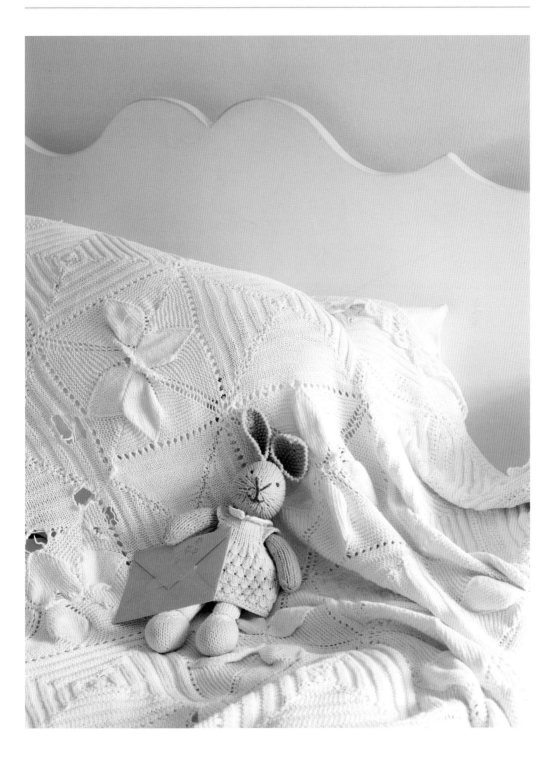

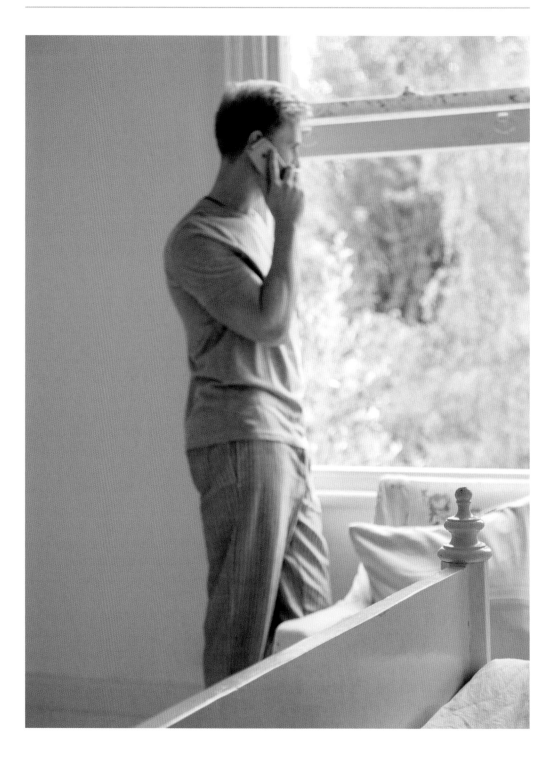

CALL A FRIEND

Call a close friend for a catch-up.

This health snack sounds remarkably simple, but it's amazing how little we do it. Back in the days when our brains were evolving we would connect with our friends every evening over the campfire. These days, we tend to see them only once in a while. One common complaint I hear in my clinic is that, especially when middle age and kids come along, connection with friends who might have been part of our lives for ten or twenty years can easily vanish. We see these people, who matter so much to us, sometimes once or twice a month at best, or sometimes once or twice a year.

Connecting with friends is something to do regularly and, ideally, on a daily basis. For this health snack, I want you to call a friend and have a chat, a giggle, or a catch-up. Remember, this isn't about calling because you have to; it's about calling because you want to. It's got to be warm and fun.

 Listen to a thought-provoking conversation about the importance of friendship on my *Feel Better, Live More* podcast at drchatterjee.com/friendship

THE LOCAL CAFÉ

Sit and enjoy your coffee while chatting to locals.

If you regularly stop off to buy coffee each morning, or have the opportunity to, perhaps you could grab yourself five minutes of connection time. Instead of ordering to-go, enjoy your drink while sitting in. Use the time to strike up a conversation with other regulars.

When I used to pop into my local café every day before work, I would bump into the same people and end up chatting to them for a few minutes every morning. It would be a great way to start each day and it soon became something that I really looked forward to.

It doesn't have to be a café, of course; it could be any social space you attend regularly.

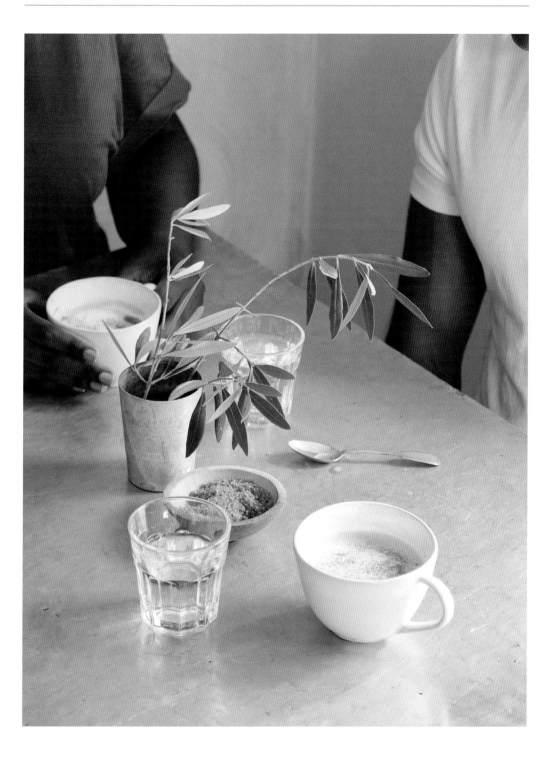

CASE STUDY

Last summer, a patient of mine, Brian, told me he was worried that he and his wife were no longer having much sex. Their relationship was otherwise fine and they were still attracted to each other, but somehow it just never seemed to happen. This was having a negative effect on his mood. When we dug into what was going on in their daily lives, I heard a story that comes up time and time again in my clinic.

I love modern technology as much as the next person. One of the many problems it creates for us, however, is that it's become so efficient at entertaining us and giving us exactly what we want, our poor human partners can't compete. Part of the change has been the extent to which tech platforms are able to get to know us personally and recommend the next news story or YouTube channel or Netflix film with such accuracy. This means we can jump into a world of fun and distraction that's been designed specifically for us wherever and whenever we like. Brian and his wife would arrive home from work, get on their laptop or tablet, then disappear into their individually curated digital worlds. The same thing is happening to couples all over the world. My wife and I are often guilty of it. When we're with the people we love, we're often not present any more.

I suggested that he and his wife get into the habit of doing a short Tea Ritual every evening. The next time he was in the city he bought a special teapot and some beautiful little Japanese cups and splashed out on some good mint tea. After dinner he and his wife would clean the kitchen, stack the dishwasher and then sit together, prepare and drink the tea, and just chat, face to face. No devices, no radio, no TV, just him and her together in the quiet.

It was only when they started their Tea Ritual that they realized how little quality time they'd been spending together. "It was almost as if we had to get to know each other all over again," he told me. Once they started talking to each other and asking how each other's day had been, they connected more, then started teasing and flirting with each other in a way they hadn't done since before the kids came along. Their relationship became romantic again and then more sexual. Soon, a beautiful Ripple Effect (page 25) began to transform other areas of their life. They were more focused at work, less reactive with their children and happier in themselves and their marriage. And it all started with that little cup of mint tea.

FORGIVE

We all feel wounded by the behavior of others at one time or another. There's not one of us who hasn't felt hurt or let down by perhaps some of the most precious people in our life. The problem for our health comes when we carry this pain around inside us, refusing to process it or let it go. It's been said that not forgiving others and holding on to resentment is like taking poison and waiting for the other person to die. I couldn't agree more.

It's no coincidence that some of the world's major religions encourage forgiveness. What our ancestors knew intuitively is now being confirmed by modern science. Research shows that an inability to forgive can increase our stress levels, reduce the quality of our sleep, affect our relationships and raise blood pressure. I've seen these processes play out many times in my consultation room. I remember one patient who was suffering from pain all over her body. She'd seen countless specialists and taken multiple painkillers, all with limited success. It was only when she started a regular practice of forgiveness that her pain really started to ease off. Carrying around the psychological pain of resentment can cause you to feel physical pain.

It's easy to underestimate the value of forgiving even the little things that happen in our daily lives. Please don't fall into this trap—these negative emotions quietly eat away at us and are corrosive for our health. Forgiving others is not about doing them a favour or letting them off the hook. It's not about saying you're fine with what they've done or being a doormat. It's *all* about you. I'd like to free and empower you by helping you to finally let that pain go.

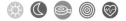

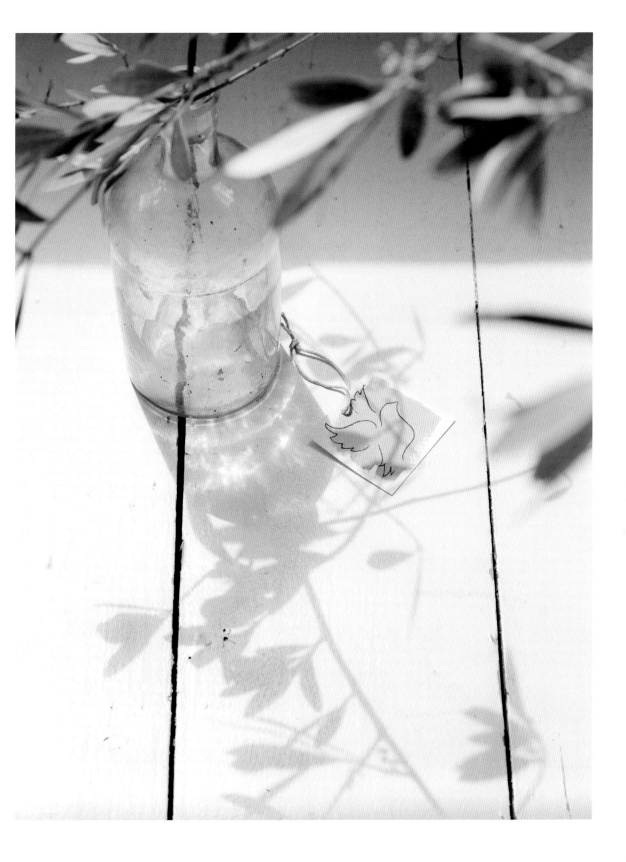

THE FORGIVENESS PRACTICE

Process your resentment by following these steps.

All of us have someone in our lives who we could do with forgiving. This health snack has been designed to set you free from the negative emotions you may have been carrying. Forgiveness is a skill which you can learn and get better at, just like anything else. The more you do it, the easier it becomes. My top tip is to start off with forgiving the small things and, over time, you will feel ready to move on to the big ones.

Sadly, some of you may have experienced significant trauma in your life. If this applies to you, these two forgiveness exercises are not appropriate. I would highly recommend you seek out a qualified professional to help you process your emotions.

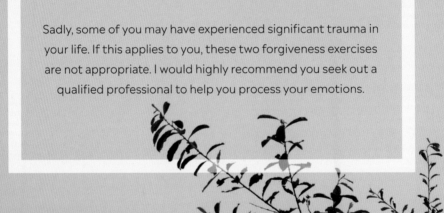

- Find a quiet space and think about who it is you want to forgive. Choose one specific incident that you feel ready to work on.

- Close your eyes and try really hard to connect with how that act made you feel. Don't rush this. It is really important to fully revisit this feeling. These feelings can be physical as well as emotional. We store and experience many powerful emotions in our bodies, yet we're often so disconnected from our physical selves that we don't notice them. For example, many of us hold tension and stress in our shoulders or lower back.

- Try to look at the situation from the other person's perspective. Put yourself in their shoes. Is there anything you can learn from doing so? What might have been going on in their life at that time to cause them to behave in that way? For example, is the work colleague who shouted at you this morning having relationship issues? Was their daughter up all night with a cold? Could they be having a tough time paying their mortgage or credit-card bill? Consider whether you may have played a role in what happened? Imagine the possibilities.

- Try to forgive them. There are many ways of doing this. Some people can simply let the feelings go once they've looked at the situation from the other person's perspective. Others imagine themselves giving the person a hug.

- See if you can start feeling any love or compassion towards them, while accepting that we all have issues in our lives and none of us is perfect.

- If the negative emotions are still there once you have finished, revisit the same incident on your next Feel Better Day. Remember, this *is* a process, not a one-off event. It may take some time.

It is very hard to give an exact time frame for the duration of this exercise. Sometimes it may take you longer than 5 minutes. It is very important that you work your way through to the end of the exercise and not stop halfway.

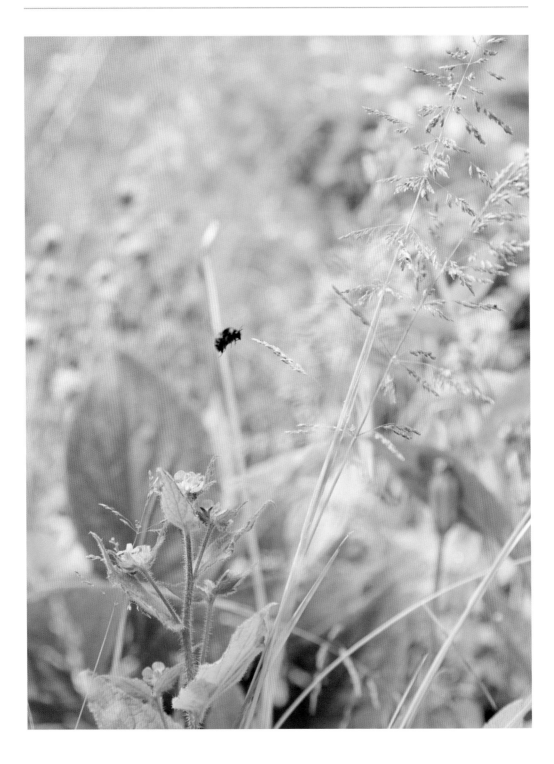

THE FORGIVENESS AFFIRMATION

Answer these four questions to help you let go of resentment.

This is a writing exercise, and some of my patients find it easier than The Forgiveness Practice (page 228). It's based around an affirmation, which is a short statement about an intention you have. More and more research is showing that affirmations can be an effective way of changing how we feel. On a new sheet of paper or in a journal, address the following four areas:

1 **Who and what are you ready to forgive?**
E.g., "I am ready to forgive the driver who swore aggressively at me this morning."

2 **How did it make you feel?**
Take some time to explore the full range of your emotions. E.g., "I felt upset, scared, angry, frustrated, and humiliated."

3 **Why are you doing this and what benefits will you receive?**
E.g., "I will feel calmer. I will feel lighter. I will feel happier. I will feel less stressed."

4 **What might have led the other person to behave in the way that they did?**
E.g., "Had they underslept? Could their child be getting bullied at school?"

Forgiveness Affirmation: Once you have answered these four questions, write down your forgiveness affirmation. E.g., "I forgive the driver and now I feel calm."

After you've written down your affirmation, say it out loud several times if you feel able to. If not, repeat it under your breath. Say it as many times as it takes to really connect with the feeling. It's quite possible that over the following days, intense emotions start to bubble up. If this happens, you may find it helpful to revisit the exercise again. Remember, for most of us, forgiveness is a process, not a one-off event. Again, it is very important that you work your way through to the end of the exercise, and not stop halfway.

If the two forgiveness exercises above bring up negative emotions that you are finding hard to manage, I would highly encourage you to seek out professional help.

CASE STUDY

Terri had been suffering from high blood pressure. She was in her early forties, a divorcee, and always seemed quite wound up and angry. If ever we were running a bit late at the clinic, she'd always find a way of letting her displeasure be known. She was the sort of person who feels the world's against them and was pretty judgemental about other people, as well as herself.

I spent quite a bit of time with Terri as I wanted to understand a bit more about why she was always so negative. After I'd seen her a few times I realized that our conversations kept coming back to her ex-husband, who'd cheated on her. I was concerned that, even though they'd divorced eight years ago, she hadn't managed to process what had happened and still held a lot of resentment about it.

Meanwhile, I was suggesting various lifestyle modifications to help deal with her blood pressure to see if I could avoid prescribing her medication. I had suggested some changes to her diet, and asked her to try reducing her alcohol intake and to go to bed a little earlier rather than staying up late each night commenting on Facebook. The problem was, I couldn't get her to engage with any of my suggestions. Whatever she tried, there always seemed to be some problem with it that made her throw her hands up in irritation. Before long I realized that, in order to help her, I would have to change my approach.

I decided to tell her about some of the research out there around forgiveness and explained that holding on to resentment might be affecting her physical health. She gave me a sharp look. "Are you talking about my ex-husband? I'm not going to forgive him for what he did. Why should I?"

I explained to her that the anger she felt towards her ex-husband was not hurting him but it was hurting her. I recommended that she see a therapist but she was reluctant, so I taught her a short exercise.

Forgiveness is hard, so to ease Terri in I started off with really simple things. I asked her to think about the last thing that annoyed her at work.

"Annoyed me?" She thought for a second.

"Well, a colleague passed me in the corridor yesterday and didn't even acknowledge me. He walked straight past me without saying a word. I was stewing on it all day."

I suggested she try The Forgiveness Practice (page 228) and reflect on what had happened at work. To her credit, Terri sincerely tried the exercise. Six weeks later, she told me she felt ready to begin the process of forgiving her ex-husband. It took several more weeks of work, but when I next checked her blood pressure it had started to come down.

Practicing forgiveness had started off a classic Ripple Effect. She told me that because she was feeling happier in herself she felt less of a need to drink so much every evening and stay up late arguing on Facebook. She had still not got round to changing her diet but planned to make a start in the coming weeks.

When I last saw her she was easy-going, bubbly, and relaxed and her blood pressure was in the normal range. She was like a different person. It was truly wonderful to see.

CELEBRATE

Life is brilliant. For most of us, it's absolutely jam-packed with tiny moments of joy and small victories. Of course, it very often doesn't feel this way. But even when it seems like we've not had the best of days, I guarantee that good things *have* happened. If you're not fully conscious of them all, it's because the brain is a problem solver. We ruminate on the things that have gone wrong because we need to learn from our mistakes. We worry about potential snags that might lie up ahead so we can plan and be prepared for them. But paying so much attention to the negative can give us a tremendously distorted view of how our lives are actually going.

There's a simple and effective way out of this trap. It involves spending five minutes a day on each of your Feel Better Days working on positive-mindset techniques. This might mean nudging yourself into feeling grateful for the little wins that have happened in an otherwise gruelling day or reframing some of the stressful things that might have occurred so that you see the silver lining. It might mean celebrating yourself and working on firming up your self-esteem.

Positive-thinking practices don't cost any money, nor do they take up much time. But the benefits are profound. Gratitude practices alone have been shown to improve physical and psychological health, to enhance sleep, and to improve self-esteem and mental resilience.

By making a regular practice of celebration you'll start to program your brain to look out for all the positives in life, the things that make it worth living. You'll find yourself noticing these moments more often and feeling grateful, encouraged and more confident. By changing the way you experience your daily life, you'll soon start to change yourself.

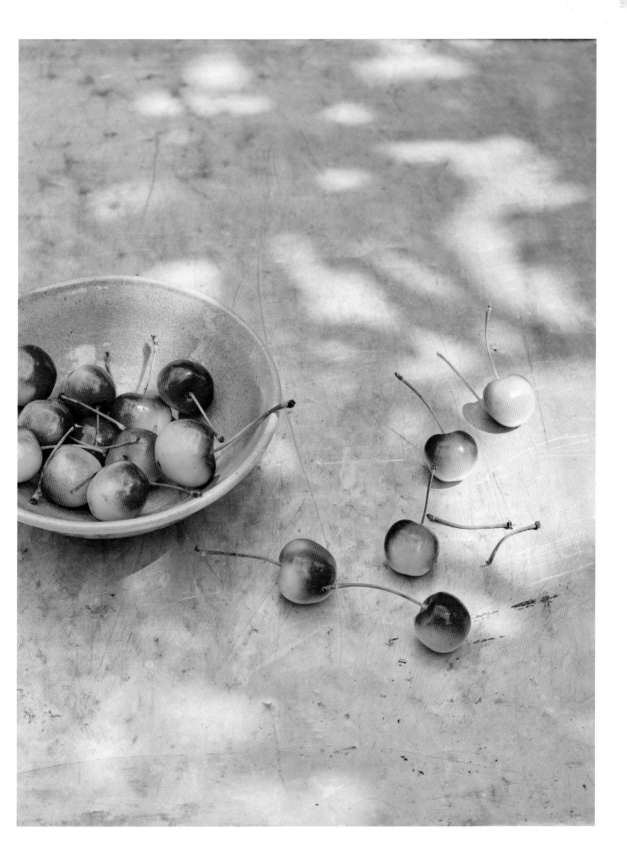

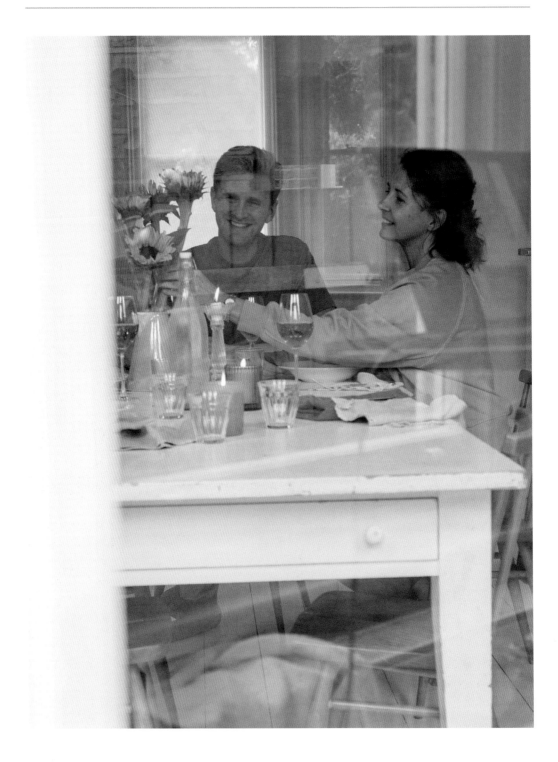

THE GRATITUDE GAME

Answer five simple questions about your day.

This is the game I play around the dinner table each night with my family. Each of us—my wife, myself, and our two children—has to answer the following five questions.

(This game used to have only three questions but over the past two years each of my kids has introduced a new one!)

- What have you done today to make someone else happy?

- What has someone else done today to make you happy?

- What have you learned today?

- What have you done today to make yourself happy?

- How did you feel when you made someone else happy?

This is a simple game that has become part and parcel of our daily family life. It helps us all focus our attention away from the negative towards the positive things that happen in our lives each day. Recently, my daughter said that one of her friends at school had made her happy as she held the door open for her because she was carrying some books. For me, I feel as if I am helping my kids cultivate a really important life skill that will help them immeasurably as they get older and begin to be exposed to many of the stresses in the modern world.

It has the added benefit of connecting us all to each other in a positive and meaningful way, going beyond the usual dreaded "So what did you do at school today?" We end up finding out things about each other that would have been unlikely to have come up in regular conversation.

This game is not just for those with families, of course. It works just as well with friends, partners, or even by yourself.

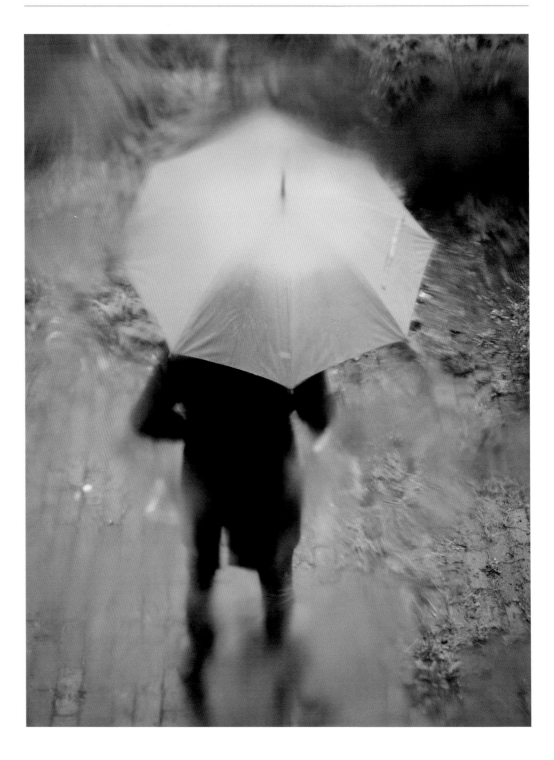

GRATITUDE FOR LIFE

Write down five things you are grateful for in your life.

I love this health snack because it's just so simple. I'd like you to spend five minutes trying to write down five things you're grateful for in your life. It could be anything at all, from the nice weather to the fact that you have a roof over your head, a job, or that you can afford to buy food each day. It could even be a tiny thing, like a particularly good episode of TV you enjoyed last night.

If you're struggling to think of anything, try using some of these ideas to guide your thoughts.

- I'm grateful that I have enough money to feed myself and my family.

- I'm grateful that I have a raincoat that kept me dry as I walked into town this morning.

- I'm grateful that I have a partner with whom I can share my experiences and worries.

- I'm grateful I have a job.

- I'm grateful for the setbacks in my life that were painful at the time but allowed me to learn and grow.

- I'm grateful to be alive and have a heart that beats thousands of times a day to keep me alive.

You could focus on some of the things you are proudest of. It could be your role as a parent, your degree, the fact that you've successfully held down a job for the past few years, or do park runs or Couch to 5K. It could simply be that, despite being tired and exhausted, you still managed to cook up a nourishing meal instead of giving in to temptation and ordering take-out.

Another way to do this exercise might be to write down five things that have given you pleasure over the last twenty-four hours. Perhaps you listened to an awesome podcast on the way to work. Perhaps your daughter or son smiled at you at just the right moment. Perhaps you watched a YouTube video that had you in stitches. Perhaps you gave your friend a lift into work. For every scenario, write down why it made you feel good and take a moment to enjoy revisiting it in your mind. Don't worry if you don't come up with five. Stop and think about each one in turn. Then, the next day, pick up where you left off.

Some of my patients enjoy doing the same exercise every day, but others love a bit of variety. It can be fun to change things up and write about different categories on each Feel Better Day. You can choose any category you like, but here are some options to get you started.

1. **Relationships**

2. **Finances**

3. **Experiences**

4. **Health**

5. **Future events**

With a bit of practice, you will soon be able to locate five things that happened to you in the last twenty-four hours that you feel grateful for. This is the most effective way of doing this health snack, as it's a regular reminder that, no matter how hard life can become, there are usually good things happening to us, even if they're not immediately apparent.

Your brain's always responding to the information it's being fed. If we start regularly feeding our brains positive information, our minds will start to become more positive.

 Listen to more about the benefits of gratitude in my conversations with Matt Haig and Rupy Aujla on my *Feel Better, Live More* podcast at drchatterjee.com/61 and drchatterjee.com/rupyaujla

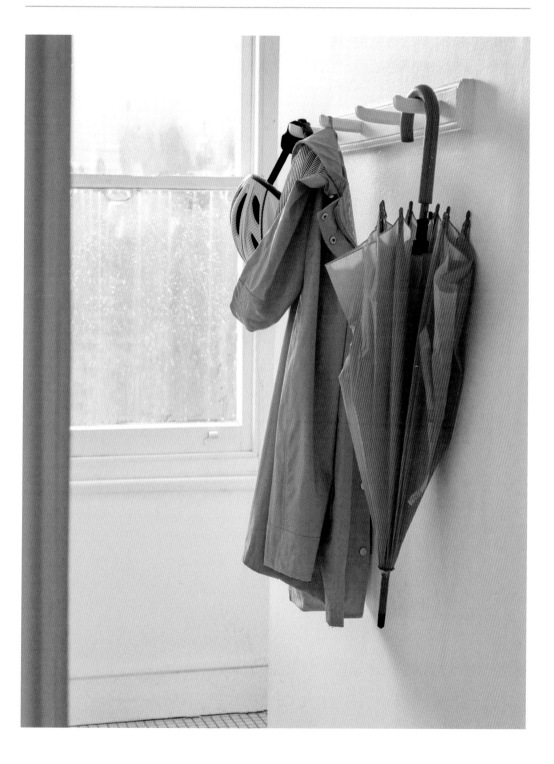

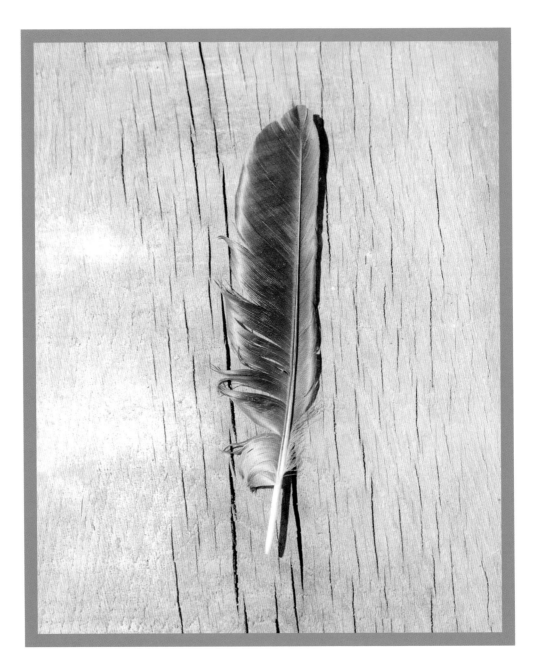

THREE TIPS FOR PRACTICING GRATITUDE

BE SPECIFIC.

The more specific you are about the things you feel grateful for, the more effective this health snack will be. For example, if you want to celebrate the fact that the barista at Starbucks made you an excellent coffee and treated you well, really drill down into the details of what was so lovely about it. What was it about the coffee they did so well? Was it the taste? How did it taste? Did they remember your name? Did they offer you a genuine smile? How did that make you feel?

FOCUS ON PEOPLE RATHER THAN THINGS.

For example, I am grateful to have my friend Philip in my life because he supports me and wants the best for me. This will generate more positive feelings than being grateful for a new pair of shoes.

CONNECT WITH YOUR EMOTIONS.

When you're writing your list, try to really experience the positive feelings the exercise is pulling out of you.

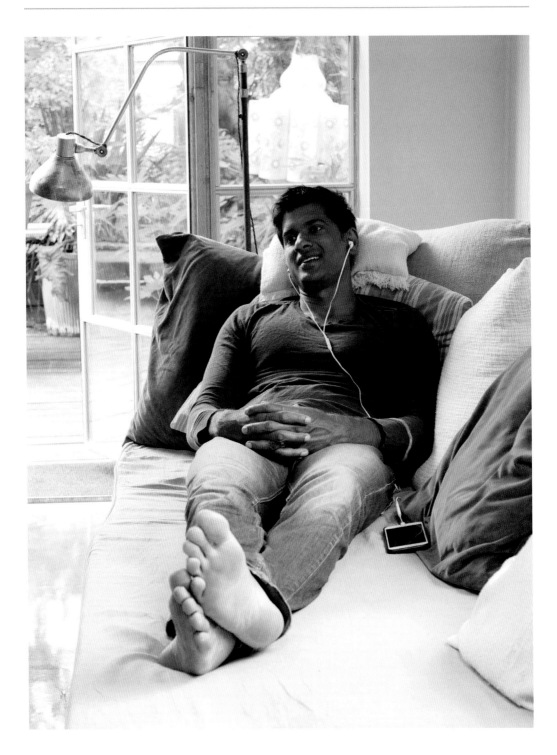

DAILY PLEASURE

Do something you love for just five minutes each day.

Life becomes even better when we do things that make us feel good. Better still, research has shown that regular doses of pleasure make us more resilient to stress. The problem is, we're often so focused on all the little problems we're facing in the immediate future that opportunities for pleasurable experiences just pass us by.

This health snack is super simple. All you have to do is spend five minutes a day intentionally doing something you love. This could be anything at all—listening to a favorite song with your eyes closed, reading a treasured book, going for a walk, or watching a funny video online. I want you to give a daily dose of pleasure the same priority you would give to eating a healthy meal.

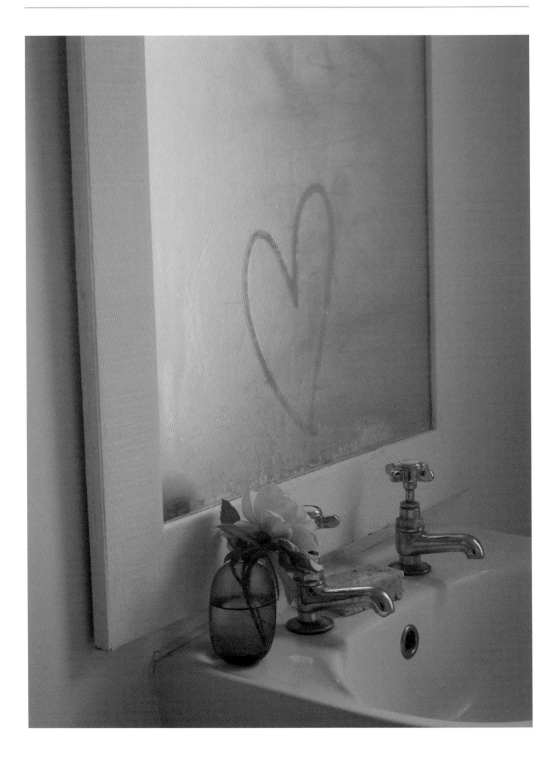

CELEBRATE YOURSELF

Write down the qualities you love about yourself.

How is your relationship with yourself? It's not even a question we typically ask ourselves. We spend our days looking outwards, thinking outwards, and caring outwards. We don't often peer back inwards and reflect on how we're doing with us.

It's extremely important that our relationship with our own selves is healthy. By "healthy," I don't mean that we're always completely uncritical of ourselves and refuse to accept any criticism from others. This isn't about arrogance or self-obsession. It's about being our own best friend. True friends aren't the ones who tell you everything you do is perfect. They're the ones who gently and caringly let you know when you've made mistakes. They genuinely want you to feel safe, happy, and successful. This is the relationship I'd like you to practice with yourself.

This health snack will help you to be the best friend you've always dreamed of. If your first thought when considering it is "I haven't got time for all that!" then you're exactly the kind of person who needs to celebrate yourself the most.

Write down as many things you love about yourself as you can think of in five minutes. This isn't as easy as it sounds, especially if you're the kind of person who's often quite harsh on yourself. If you find it hard at first, think about what others would say if they were asked to list your positive qualities.

 Listen to a beautiful conversation with the hypnotherapist Chloe Brotheridge about the importance of celebrating yourself on my *Feel Better, Live More* podcast at drchatterjee. com/bravenewgirl

CELEBRATE OTHERS

Write a letter to someone who has done something good for you.

Another way to enjoy all the benefits of gratitude is to write a letter to someone you love or value. Think about someone who has done something good for you. It could be a small favor or a compliment paid to you in the last week or so, or it could be something bigger from your more distant past. It could be your parent, a friend, a work colleague, a parent from the school run, or the clerk at your local train station. Take up to five minutes to address this person in a letter. Let them know what they've done and how it made you feel. Tell them how their behavior affected your life or changed the way you think.

For example, you could write a letter to the ticket officer at your local station and thank them for giving you the information that enabled you to purchase a cheaper fare. Write down the joy you felt and how much you appreciated it.

When you've written the letter, simply think about this memory, focusing on your feelings of gratitude. You can amplify the benefit of this health snack massively by actually giving this person the letter or writing it into an email. Alternatively, if you don't feel able to do this, you could write your gratitude letters and store them in a box or a folder. This could act as a powerful gratitude battery you could use to charge yourself up with when you're feeling lonely or down.

The benefits to your health come from the actual writing of the letter. Whether you give someone the letter or simply write it is up to you.

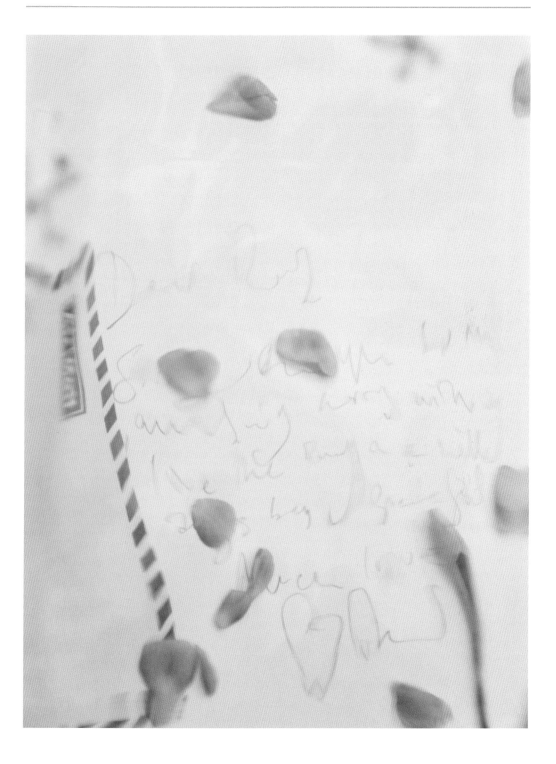

REFRAME THE MOMENT

Practice being kind to yourself by reframing something from your day.

This health snack involves thinking about something you did during the day (or the previous day, if you're doing this in the morning) that you might have done differently, reframing it, and letting go of self-blame.

When we regret our actions, it's easy to snap into a blameful state of mind, cursing ourselves and calling ourselves out. I'd like you to calmly and compassionately ask why you behaved the way you did. Did you fall out with a work colleague because you stayed up late last night binge-watching a box set and consequently woke up feeling tired and irritable? Did you shout at your kids because you'd just opened an unwelcome bill? Did you have a fight with your partner because you'd just looked in the mirror and didn't like your appearance?

This process of reflecting back and reviewing what happened each day is incredibly useful. It gives you the opportunity to take a breath and be kind to yourself. Psychologists believe that this exercise is much more powerful when you write it down. There's something about the process of physically noting your train of thought that makes it real and powerful. It just doesn't seem to happen in the same way if it stays inside our heads.

I'd like you to sit in front of a fresh piece of paper or a journal for five minutes and work through the following questions.

- Which moment from the last twenty-four hours would you like to reframe? Write down a simple description of what happened, as if you were an observer.

- What's the worst interpretation of your behavior? What would your harshest critic tell you your behavior shows about who you are?

List five reasons why this viewpoint is wrong.

When you've finished, write: "I forgive myself for . . . ," adding in the moment you've been working through. Once you've written it down, allow yourself a few moments to really focus on the statement, experiencing all the emotions it brings.

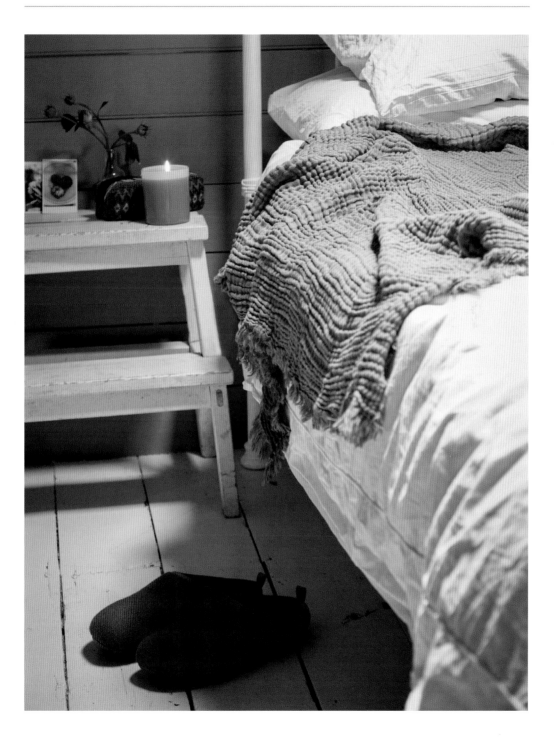

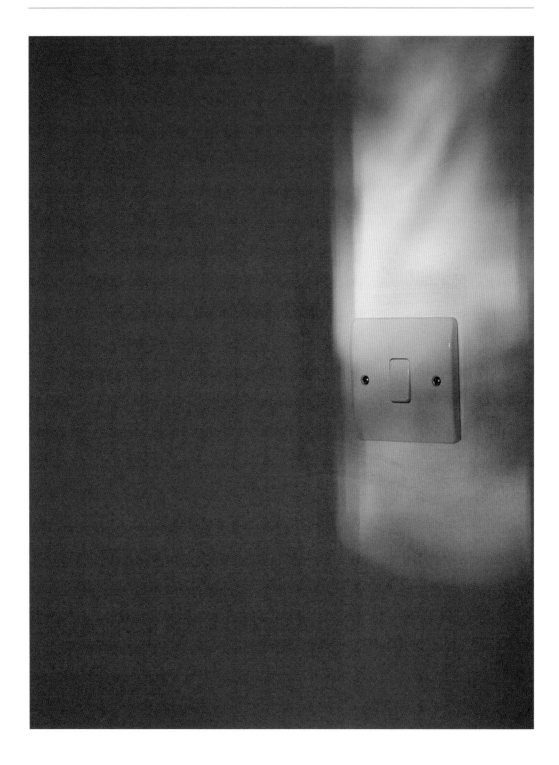

REFRAME THE DAY

Write down three things that went well for you today.

This is an incredibly powerful exercise that research has shown to increase people's happiness immediately, with the positive effects in some people still present six months later.

Write down three things that went well for you today. Here are some suggestions.

- Did someone make you a cup of tea at work?

- Did someone let you turn out of a side street on to a main road?

- Did someone offer you their seat on the bus?

- Did someone tell you that your backpack was open and that things may fall out?

- Did your partner tidy the house before you came home?

After each act write a sentence saying why the positive event happened and what it tells you about the world. It could be that your colleague made you a hot drink because they care about you, or the driver let you turn out of the side street because there are good, caring people everywhere.

If this practice feels tricky at first, don't worry. That's perfectly normal. The more you do it, the better at it you'll become. The simple process of pausing and reflecting on these positive events can be incredibly beneficial, changing how you see the world around you.

REFRAME THE FUTURE

The idea that we might "reframe the future" sounds impossible. But it really is true.

It involves saying an affirmation. As discussed in The Forgiveness Affirmation on page 231, affirmations are short, powerful statements that feed your brain positive information. So, think: what kind of person do you wish to be today? Would you like to be compassionate and patient? Calm and happy? Patient and forgiving? Choose your affirmation and write it down. It must be in the present tense. For example, "I am calm and happy" or "I am patient and forgiving."

Say your affirmation out loud, or under your breath. Some people prefer to do this with their eyes closed. Repeat it continuously for as long as you can, but for at least one minute. I appreciate that you may find it challenging to do this for a whole 5 minutes. That is completely fine. Even 1–2 minutes of this can be incredibly helpful. If you choose to keep your eyes closed and repeat it under your breath, it can feel like a calming, meditative practice.

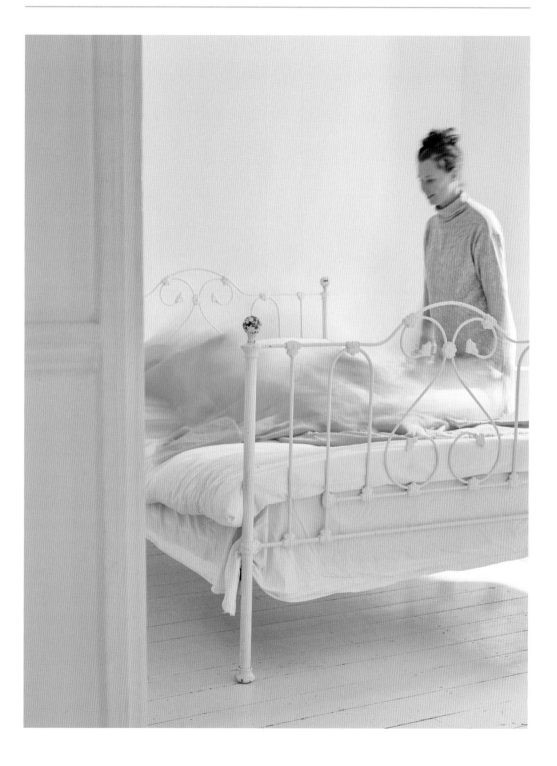

MAKING IT STICK

This is the last time I'm going to mention this, I promise! As with all the *Feel Better in 5* health snacks, it really is important to attach them to an existing part of your daily routine. I do my own gratitude practice at the dinner table with my family, which means I don't need to find any extra time in my day to do it. It's now become a habit, and I miss it on the occasions when I can't join in because I'm away. Within weeks of starting to do it, it became an automatic behavior that just happens when we're all at the dinner table, without us thinking about it.

As you have already learned, another important strategy to help make new behaviors stick is to set up your environment in such a way that makes the behavior you wish to engage in as easy as possible. If you have chosen one of the writing-based health snacks, consider keeping your notebook or journal beside your bed. This also acts as a visual trigger, so that every night when you get to your bed, you are being prompted to do your health snack.

The more of these little tips you can introduce around each of your health snacks, the more likely it is that you will be doing them not just once, but day after day, week after week, year after year.

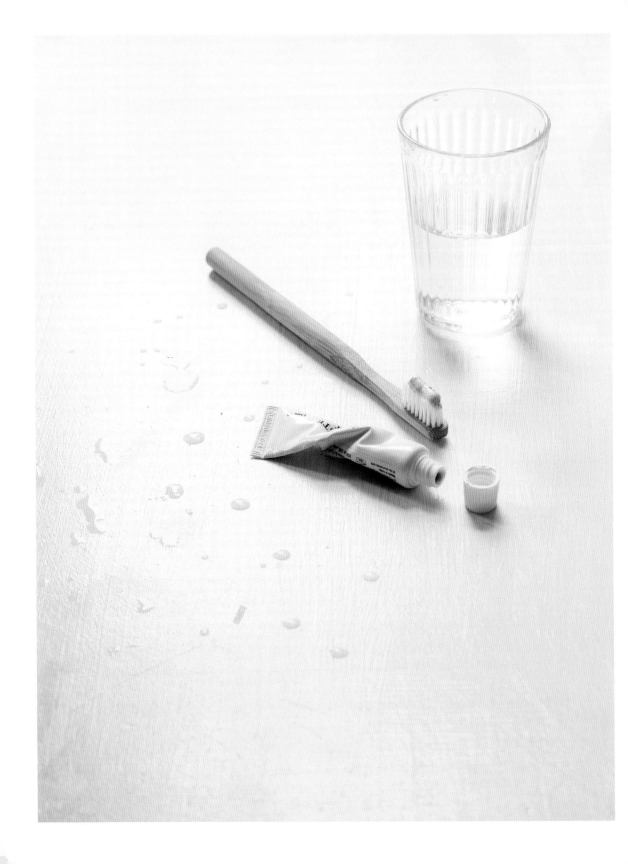

BRUSHING YOUR TEETH FOR EVERYTHING ELSE

You brush your teeth twice a day. Nobody has to remind you to do this. You don't have to gather up the energy to do it or wonder if you have an available slot in your busy schedule. You barely even think about it. The brush goes under the tap, the toothpaste slides on, and there you are, giving up the time to take fantastic care of your teeth fourteen times a week. It barely takes a thought.

Your teeth are important, of course, but the fact is that a damaged tooth is often far easier to fix than a damaged heart, a damaged insulin system, a damaged back, or a damaged relationship with your partner or children. And yet so many of us don't give these other critical parts of our mental and physical wellbeing anywhere near the attention we give our teeth.

If I have one overriding mission in life, it's to see that change. The health snacks in this book have been designed to be simple and easy, just like brushing your teeth. But make no mistake, they're also underpinned by cutting-edge science and my two decades of practice as a doctor. They'll have biological effects on your body, mood-enhancing effects on your mind, and a nourishing effect on your heart.

Just like brushing your teeth, their secret is that they don't take much effort or time. They work because they're done little and often. It's the repetition that makes them powerful. It's the drip-drip-drip effect, not the big, occasional push, that will slowly but surely transform your health. Just as one cigarette won't kill you, one health snack won't cure you. But the more you do, the more you'll inevitably alter your body and mind for the better.

It's never too late to change your habits. Whether you're in your twenties or your seventies, *Feel Better in 5* will work for you. Once three regular health snacks have become a part of your *Feel Better in 5* routine and seem virtually effortless, you'll probably want to build on them. Feel free to add snacks, or lengthen the time you take to do them, or start to do them seven days a week, all of which will increase their power.

But if you're happy sticking with the three snacks five times a week, that's OK, too. You'll still experience huge benefits. The behavior-change expert James Clear compares the effect of adding these small habits to your daily routine to changing the route of an airplane heading from Los Angeles to New York by a tiny 3.5 degrees. "You will land in Washington, D.C., instead of New York," he writes in his book *Atomic Habits*. "Such a small change is barely noticeable at takeoff—the nose of the airplane moves just a few feet—but when magnified across the entire United States, you end up hundreds of miles apart." The same is true of your health. If all you do is five minutes of journalling, five minutes of bodyweight exercises, and five minutes of gratitude on each of your Feel Better Days, your life will change for the better. By the end of the first month, you'll be a different person. You'll be happier, calmer, stronger, and healthier, and have better self-esteem. From just fifteen minutes a day.

You've bought this book because you're ready to become a new you. You've seen what it takes and how simple it is. You can no longer tell yourself you're too busy. You can no longer tell yourself it's too difficult. You can no longer tell yourself that nothing ever works. All your excuses are gone. Nobody can tell me they don't have fifteen minutes a day to spend on themselves. If this isn't the moment you finally change your journey, when is that moment going to be? Don't put off doing your first health snack until tomorrow.

DO IT NOW!

STILL FEEL YOU
DON'T HAVE TIME?

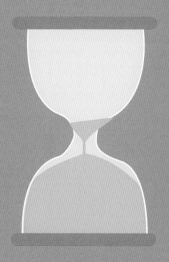

IF THIS ISN'T THE MOMENT YOU FINALLY
CHANGE YOUR JOURNEY, WHEN IS THAT MOMENT
GOING TO BE?

CHART YOUR SUCCESS

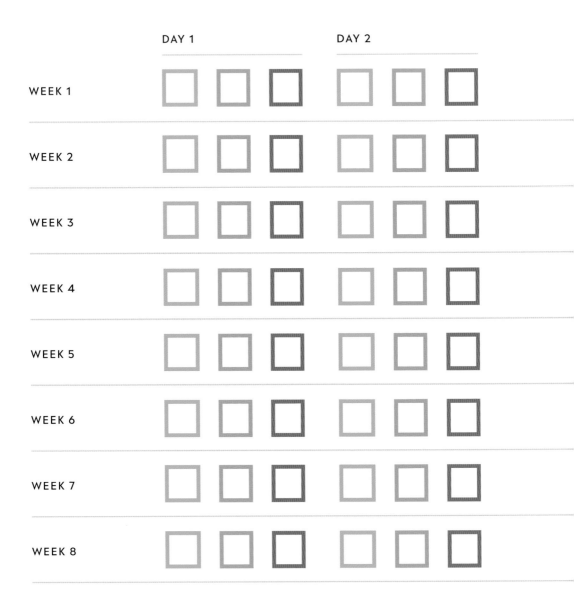

	DAY 1			DAY 2		
WEEK 1	☐	☐	☐	☐	☐	☐
WEEK 2	☐	☐	☐	☐	☐	☐
WEEK 3	☐	☐	☐	☐	☐	☐
WEEK 4	☐	☐	☐	☐	☐	☐
WEEK 5	☐	☐	☐	☐	☐	☐
WEEK 6	☐	☐	☐	☐	☐	☐
WEEK 7	☐	☐	☐	☐	☐	☐
WEEK 8	☐	☐	☐	☐	☐	☐

Every time you complete a health snack, mark it on the chart above. Either place a sticker in the correct box or use a pen to give yourself a check mark. You will quickly see how your successes build up and this will help you build momentum. Remember, try to feel a positive emotion every time you are completing this table.

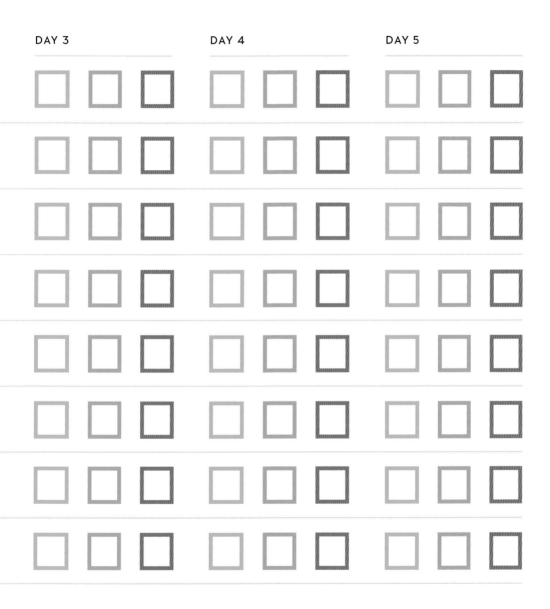

DAY 3

DAY 4

DAY 5

Once you have completed this chart, go to drchatterjee.com/wallchart to print off another one and continue tracking your successes!

FREQUENTLY ASKED QUESTIONS

What happens if I miss a day?

If you miss a day, there is no need to worry. There are two spare days per week and you can make up the missing health snacks on one of these days.

What happens if I come home from work after a busy day exhausted and don't have the time and energy to do my three health snacks?

If this happens, I would recommend that you try your best to get at least one health snack fully completed—it will only take you five minutes. This helps you to maintain momentum, which is a key ingredient in making long-term behavior change.

An alternative is to do 1–2 minutes on each of your three health snacks. Again, this will only take you a few minutes in total and helps keep up momentum. *Feel Better in 5* is about building up daily habits for life. Doing a little is better than doing nothing—in fact, spending a few minutes on your health snacks will probably make you feel less exhausted!

What if I do a health snack but don't manage the full five minutes?

If you don't manage the full five minutes, that is perfectly OK. The important thing is that you do something. Of course, I would prefer you to do the full duration of health snack but I don't want you to get into that "all or nothing" mindset. Even doing two minutes of deep breathing or two minutes of a gratitude practice will still yield benefits, and importantly, will keep up momentum.

Can I start the program off more slowly?

Absolutely. If you feel that it may be too challenging to introduce three different health snacks per day into your life in one go, I would recommend you start off at a slightly slower pace. In Week One, I would recommend that you start off by doing only one health snack on each of your Feel Better days. During this first week, try really hard to do your chosen five-minute health snack in the same place and at the same time each day. This will make it much more likely you will be able to consistently perform it.

At the start of Week Two, add in your second health snack from a different menu. For example, if your first health snack was from Mind, then choose a health snack from Body or Heart instead. In Week Two, you will be doing two health snacks per day. Remember, this will only take you ten minutes in total. In Week Three, add in your third health snack from a different menu, to bring you up to fifteen minutes per day.

The key to successful behavior change is to start small and slowly install new habits into your life.

Do I need to do my health snacks at different times of the day?

Absolutely not—you can personalize this program to suit your life and do your three health snacks at times that suit you and your daily routine. If you prefer, you can do all three health snacks one after the other. In fact, many of my patients like to wake up and do all three health snacks right away, as part of their morning routine. This means that within fifteen minutes of waking up, they have completed their entire program for the day!

What if I don't manage to complete all three health snacks in one day and manage only one or two?

If you only manage to complete one or two health snacks on a particular day, you will still gain benefits. If this happens, you can either double up on the one you missed the following day or make it up on one of your free days. The goal is to get those fifteen ticks, five days per week, week after week, month after month. Remember, Rome was not built in a day.

If I already go to the gym, cycle regularly or do a weekly fitness class, can I miss out the Body health snack?

If you regularly attend a health class or gym, that is fantastic. However, it is not a substitute for my *Feel Better in 5* program. This plan is about creating new daily habits. It is these daily habits that create your short-term and long-term health, NOT the once a week gym session.

A daily Body health snack will actually enhance your other movement activities. If you are already fairly active, why not choose a health snack from "Body" that works on a different aspect of your health. For example, if you run and cycle already, why not do five minutes of restorative yoga poses each day or a five-minute strength workout, like The Classic Five. One of my close friends is a keen runner and cycles to work, every day. He did not think that my program was for him, yet within two weeks of doing it, he found he could run further, cycle up hills for longer and had more energy.

When done consistently, these small daily habits will have a huge impact on your health and wellbeing.

FURTHER RESOURCES

For a more detailed look into the science behind the recommendations in *Feel Better in 5*, please take a look at my first two books, *The 4 Pillar Plan* and *The Stress Solution*.

You can also listen to in-depth conversations with leading health experts and inspirational public figures about a range of different topics (including gut health, brain health, food, sleep, movement, breathing, and so much more) on my free weekly podcast, *Feel Better, Live More*—you can find all episodes at drchatterjee.com/podcast or by searching on all podcast platforms such as Apple Podcasts, Spotify, and Acast.

My understanding of the science of behavior change has been greatly enhanced and informed by the work of some brilliant researchers. If you are interested in this area, I would highly encourage you to check out the work and books of:

- B. J. Fogg, author of *Tiny Habits*
- James Clear, author of *Atomic Habits*
- Charles Duhigg, author of *The Power of Habit*

To learn more about the science and benefits of forgiveness, I would recommend you look up Fred Luskin's work from the Stanford University Forgiveness Projects at learningtoforgive.com.

If you enjoy doing my five-minute workouts and would like more guidance on your technique and potential progressions, I would recommend you seek out the help of a personal trainer or join a local exercise class.

If you enjoy doing the five-minute restorative yoga flows and want to learn more, I would highly encourage you to join a local class with a qualified yoga instructor. This will help you improve your technique and learn new progressions that you can introduce into your daily "Restore" health snack. For those of you who prefer to learn online, I would recommend you look up the YouTube channel "Yoga with Adriene."

If you are interested in learning more about the innovative movements in "Balance" that are designed to wake up your body and get it moving more efficiently, I would encourage you to look at Gary Ward's "Wake Your Body Up" and "Wake Your Feet Up" online series, at www.findingcentre.co.uk.

If you have enjoyed this book, you may enjoy keeping up to date with my latest work by receiving my free weekly e-mail newsletter. My subscribers are the first to hear about any new articles that I have written, new projects that I am working on, my latest podcasts, and new books that I am writing. In addition, I regularly send out information on books and articles that I have come across that I think you would find helpful.

You can sign up and join my online community at drchatterjee.com/subscribe.

ACKNOWLEDGMENTS

As I look back now on another completed manuscript (my third one in three years!), I must admit that I am not quite sure how I got here. One thing is for certain: this book would never have been written without the help and support of a long list of people. Throughout my life, I have been incredibly fortunate to have had a supportive family, inspiring mentors, and a close group of remarkable friends.

First and foremost, I would like to thank my wife, Vidhaata. She has shown incredible patience as my seemingly endless book-writing has eaten into evenings, weekends, and holidays. She has also played every conceivable role in the writing of this book including researcher, critic, sounding board, and editor. This book would not have been the same without her.

Jainam and Anoushka, you both inspire me every day. Thanks for being patient while Daddy finished writing and thanks for all your suggestions and helping me come up with new ideas. You teach me what life is truly about on a daily basis and I love you both more than words can say. I hope this book makes you proud and helps to create a healthier and happier society for you to grow up in.

Mum and Dada, thank you for always believing in me in every single project that I undertake.

Chetana and Dinesh, thank you for the gift of having two more parents.

I am lucky to have an incredible group of close friends who endlessly listen to my new ideas, provide creative input, and challenge me to be the best that I can. A heartfelt thank you to Will Storr, Luke Fisher, Jeremy Hawkey, Ayan Panja, Phil Creswell, Jodie Hawkey, Michael Ash, Antony Haynes, Carron Scrimgeour, Steve Lau, Bobby Chatterjee, Dhru Purohit, and Christian Platt.

Gary Ward, thanks for collaborating with me once again. I know these movement sequences will help so many people. Your work deserves to be spread all over the world.

Will Francis, you epitomize what anyone could wish for in an agent—thank you.

Clare, thanks for your dedication, versatility, and your ability to juggle multiple balls at once. I couldn't do this without you.

Jo, you have been an incredible asset and are invaluable in helping me spread my message.

Thanks also to Miguel Mateas, Bernice Hulme, Diana Davidson, Philip Owen, Sophie Laurimore, Carina Rizvi, Kirsty Gordon, Zoë Nelson, and Ellis Hazelgrove.

I am fortunate to work with what is probably the best team in publishing! A huge thank you to the phenomenal team of amazing women at Penguin Life: Venetia, Emily, Julia, Josie, Marianne, Alice, and Emma.

Miranda, Clare, and Polly—my fabulous new creative team! You have been a joy to work with and have shown phenomenal dedication and expertise to help me make this book as accessible as possible.

And, finally, thank you to every single one of my readers. Life is short and time is precious—thank you for giving me some of yours. I hope that you feel inspired and are now well equipped with new tools to start making small changes that will have a big impact on your health and happiness.

HEALTH SNACKS INDEX

1 MIND

The Brain Tap
66

The 5 Step Release
69

5 Minutes in Nature
79

5 Minutes of Flow
87

Simple Breathing
94

Breath Counting
96

Mind the Blueberries
105

Happy Brain Smoothie
106

The Gut Bugs Health
Snack
108

2 BODY

The Classic 5
119

The Power 5
136

Simple Sweat
143

The Easy Kneesy
146

The HIIT Squad
150

Just Play!
157

Dancing
159

Jumping Rope
161

Desk Jockey Workout
169

The Clock Workout
179

The Morning Wake-Up
Flow
191

Day's End Release Flow
195

3 HEART

The Love List
214

Tea Ritual
216

The Kindness Practice
218

Call a Friend
221

The Local Café
222

The Forgiveness Practice
228

The Forgiveness
Affirmation 231

The Gratitude Game
237

Gratitude for Life
239

Daily Pleasure
245

Celebrate Yourself
247

Celebrate Others
248

Reframe the Moment
250

Reframe the Day
253

Reframe the Future
254

INDEX

Abdominal Stretch 196
adult coloring books 88, 91
anger 45, 56
anxiety 45, 56, 70–71
arm spirals 169, 175
athletic performance 51, 57

back pain 45, 56, 186–7
Balance 113, 166–7
  case study 186–7
  Clock Workout 179–85
  Desk Jockey Workout 169–77
  health benefits 41
bedroom 33
behavior change, 6 tips 26–37
blood pressure 47–8, 56, 232–3
blueberries, Mind the
  Blueberries   105
Body 17, 111, 114–15
  Balance 166–87
  health benefits 41
  making it stick 204–5
  Play 154–65
  Restore 188–203
  snacks menu 112–13
  Strength 116–33
  Sweat 134–53
brain health 51, 57
Brain Tap 66
  and creativity 52
  and wellbeing 54
Breath Counting 96
  and anger 45
  and athletic performance 51
  and focus 53
Breathe 61, 92–3
  Breath Counting 96
  case study 98–9
  health benefits 41
  making it stick 100–101

Simple Breathing 94–5
burpees 150, 151

Call a Friend 221
  and wellbeing 54
Celebrate 209, 234
  Celebrate Others 248
  Celebrate Yourself 247
  Daily Pleasure 245
  Gratitude for Life 239–40
  The Gratitude Game 237
  health benefits 41
  Reframe the Day 253
  Reframe the Future 254
  Reframe the Moment 250
  three tips for practicing
  gratitude
  243
Celebrate Others 248
  and depression 46
Celebrate Yourself 247
  and back pain 45
  and excess weight 47
  and type 2 diabetes 48
chronic pain 46, 56, 98–9
The Classic 5 119–31
  and brain health 51
  and happiness 53
  and high blood pressure 48
  and longevity 54
  and type 2 diabetes 48
Clear, James 260
Clock Workout 179–85
  and athletic performance 51
  and wellbeing 54
closer relationships 51, 57,
  224–5
  see also Connect
coloring books 88, 91
Connect 209, 212–13

Call a Friend 221
case study 224–5
  health benefits 41
  The Kindness Practice 218
  The Local Café 222
  Love List 214
  Tea Ritual 216
core 115
core clock 179, 185
creativity 52, 57
crucifix 169, 176

Daily Pleasure 245
  and stress 48
Dancing 159, 164–5
  and closer relationships 51
  and creativity 52
  and depression 46
Day's End Release Flow 195–200
  and focus 53
  and gut issues 47
  and kindness to yourself 53
  and stress 48
depression 46, 56
Desk Jockey Workout 169–77,
  186–7
  and back pain 45
diabetes 48, 56
Download 61, 65
  Brain Tap 66
  case study 70–71
  5 Step Release 69
  health benefits 41
  making it stick 72–3
drawing 87

The Easy Kneesy 146–9
  and excess weight 46
energy 52, 57
environment 31–3

excess weight 46–7, 56
exercise *see* Body

family health 52, 57
Feel Better Days 39, 260
5 Minutes in Nature 79–80
  and family health 52
  and happiness 53
  and sleep 54
  and stress 48
5 Minutes of Flow 87–8
  and back pain 45
  and closer relationships 51
  and energy 52
  and headaches 47
  and longevity 54
5 Step Release 69
  and anxiety 45
Flow 61, 84
  case study 90–91
  5 Minutes of Flow 87–8
  health benefits 41
focus 53, 57
Fogg, B. J. 26
Forgive 209, 226
  case study 232–3
  The Forgiveness Affirmation 231
  The Forgiveness Practice 228–9
  health benefits 41
The Forgiveness Affirmation 231
  and chronic pain 46
  and high blood pressure 48
The Forgiveness Practice 228–9
  and anger 45
  and excess weight 47
frontal cogs 169, 173

glute bridges 119, 131
glutes 115
gratitude 234, 243
Gratitude for Life 239–40
  and brain health 51
  and focus 53

and longevity 54
The Gratitude Game 237
  and family health 52
Gut Bugs Health Snack 108
  and gut issues 47
gut issues 47, 56

habits 22–3
  changing 26–8, 259–60
hamstrings 115
happiness 53, 57
Happy Brain Smoothie 106
  and brain health 51
  and type 2 diabetes 48
headaches 47, 56
health 15–16
health journey 19–21
health snacks 16, 17, 22–3, 39, 259–60
  6 tips for making changes that stick   26–37
  Body 111–205
  health benefits 40–57
  Heart 207–257
  how to choose 42–3
  Mind 60–109
  Ripple Effect 25
  wall chart 36, 262–3
Heart 17, 207, 210–211
  Celebrate 234–54
  Connect 212–25
  Forgive 226–33
  health benefits 41
  making it stick 256–7
  snacks menu 208–9
high blood pressure 47–8, 56, 232–3
high knees with shoulder press 146
HIIT (High Intensity Interval Training) 134–5
  The Easy Kneesy 146–9
  HIIT Squad 150–53
  The Power 5 136–41
  Simple Sweat 143
  see also Sweat

jigsaw puzzles 88
jogging on the spot 136, 137
jumping jacks 136, 139
Jumping Rope 161
Just Play! 157

The Kindness Practice 218
  and happiness 53
kindness to yourself 53, 57
kitchen 31
knees 146–9
knitting 87

listening to music 88
The Local Café 222
longevity 54, 57
Love List 214
  and gut issues 47
lunge 119, 121
lunge clock 179, 181

meditation 92
  see also Breathe
Mind 17, 59, 62–3
  Breathe 92–101
  Download 65–73
  Flow 84–91
  health benefits 41
  Nature 74–83
  Nourish 102–9
  snacks menu 60–61
Mind the Blueberries 105
mindfulness 84
  see also Flow
mobile phones 33
Morning Wake-up Flow 191–2
  and chronic pain 46
  and headaches 47
mountain climbers 136, 139, 150, 153
movement *see* Body
music 88

Nature 61, 74
  case study 82–3
  5 Minutes in Nature 79–80
  health benefits 41, 76–7
Nourish 61, 102–3
  Gut Bugs Health Snack 108
  Happy Brain Smoothie 106
  health benefits 41
  Mind the Blueberries 105

pain see back pain; chronic pain
painting 87
phones 33
Pigeon Pose 198
Play 113, 154
  case study 164–5
  Dancing 159
  and family health 52
  health benefits 41
  Just Play! 157
  making it stick 162–3
  Jumping Rope 161
playing music 88
positive self-talk 34
The Power 5 136–41, 143
  and anger 45
  and sleep 54
Puppy-Dog Stretch 196
push-ups
  on knees 146, 149
  Strength 119, 127–9
  Sweat 136, 141

quads 115

reading 88
Reframe the Day 253
  and creativity 52
  and energy 52
  and sleep 54
Reframe the Future 254
  and athletic performance 51
Reframe the Moment 250
  and anxiety 45
  and headaches 47
  and kindness to yourself 53

relationships 51, 57, 224–5
  see also Connect
Restore 113, 188–9
  case study 202–3
  Day's End Release Flow
  195–200
  health benefits 41
  Morning Wake-up Flow 191–2
reverse 119, 123
Ripple Effect 25

self-talk 34
shoulder clock 179, 183
shoulder taps 150, 153
Simple Breathing 94–5
  and chronic pain 46
  and excess weight 46
  and high blood pressure 47–8
  and kindness to yourself 53
Simple Sweat 143
  and anxiety 45
  and energy 52
sitting arm punch 146, 149
sleep 54, 57
smartphones 33
smoothies
  Happy Brain Smoothie 106
  Mind the Blueberries 105
squats 119, 125
  with knee to hand 146
  squat jumps 150, 153
  sumo squats 136, 141
standing glute extension 131
straight punches 146, 149
Strength 113, 116–17
  The Classic 5 119–31
  health benefits 41
  making it stick 132–3
stress 48, 56
sumo squats 136, 141
Sweat 113, 134–5
  case study 144–5
  The Easy Kneesy 146–9
  and excess weight 46
  health benefits 41
  HIIT Squad 150–53

The Power 5 136–41
Simple Sweat 143

Tea Ritual 216, 225
  and closer relationships 51
Thread the Needle 195
Toribio-Mateas, Miguel 106
Triangle Pose 200
type 2 diabetes 48, 56

wall charts 36, 262–3
wall cogs 169, 171
Ward, Gary 167
weight 46–7, 56
wellbeing 54, 57
workouts
  Strength 116–33
  Sweat 134–53

yoga 188–9, 202–3
  Day's End Release Flow
  195–200
  Morning Wake Up Flow 191–2

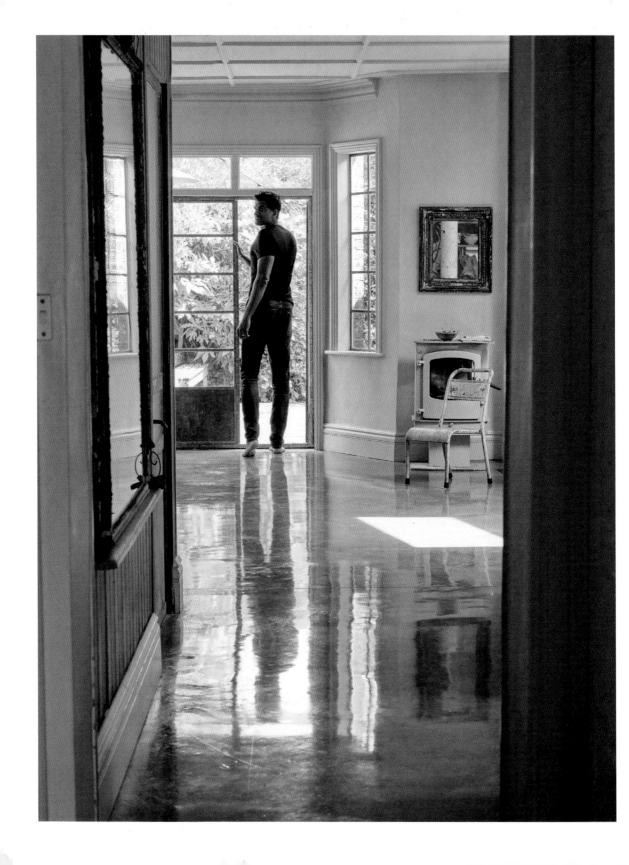